Designing Science Presentations

Designing Science Presentations

A Visual Guide to Figures, Papers, Slides, Posters, and More

Second Edition

Matt Carter

*Department of Biology, Williams College,
Williamstown, MA, United States*

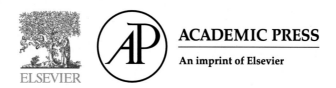

ELSEVIER

ACADEMIC PRESS

An imprint of Elsevier

Academic Press is an imprint of Elsevier
125 London Wall, London EC2Y 5AS, United Kingdom
525 B Street, Suite 1650, San Diego, CA 92101, United States
50 Hampshire Street, 5th Floor, Cambridge, MA 02139, United States
The Boulevard, Langford Lane, Kidlington, Oxford OX5 1GB, United Kingdom

Library of Congress Cataloging-in-Publication Data
A catalog record for this book is available from the Library of Congress

British Library Cataloguing-in-Publication Data
A catalogue record for this book is available from the British Library

ISBN: 978-0-12-815377-2

For information on all Academic Press publications visit our
website at https://www.elsevier.com/books-and-journals

Publisher: Nikki Levy
Acquisitions Editor: Natalie Farra
Editorial Project Manager: Tracy I. Tufaga
Production Project Manager: Maria Bernard
Cover Designer: Mark Rogers

Typeset by TNQ Technologies

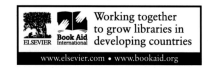

Working together
to grow libraries in
developing countries

www.elsevier.com • www.bookaid.org

Contents

Contents

About the author

Matt Carter is Associate Professor of Biology at Williams College where he teaches courses in neuroscience and physiology. His research focuses on how the brain regulates food intake and sleep. In addition to publishing articles and presenting talks on his research, he also enjoys giving workshops on scientific presentation design. He is a recipient of the Walter Gores Award for Excellence in Teaching from Stanford University and the Nelson Bushnell Prize for Teaching and Writing from Williams College. He lives in Williamstown with his wife and three children.

Acknowledgments

Writing a book about science presentation design may unintentionally misconvey that I think I know better than others. In reality, it is *because* of others that I learned all of the principles in this book. My mentors, colleagues, friends, and family—both in and out of science—taught me all I know. Indeed, I found myself smiling while writing and editing many of the pages in this book because I remembered the exact moments when I learned specific skills from my colleagues. I especially found myself smiling while writing and editing the second edition of this book because many of my colleagues gave me very helpful, insightful feedback. Thanks to everyone for helping me grow.

First and foremost, I thank my family for allowing me to be a bit mentally distracted while I put this second edition together. I cannot adequately articulate my appreciation for my wife, Ali, for all the support she provides me every day. Ali is my best friend, and I am so thankful for her calm, her wisdom, and her support. She is the rock of our family… which has grown over the years. When I finished the first edition of this book, our son, Liam, was 2 years old—now he is 10, our daughter Hadley is 6, and our other daughter Sadie is a year-and-a-half old. I love all of you so much.

Both of my parents enjoyed science and writing, and their passions in life greatly influenced me. Mom, thanks for sharing your joy of learning and for teaching me the value of hard work. Dad, thanks for sending me cool science stories from all disciplines and teaching me that good writing is really good editing. And thanks to my brothers, Josh and Stephen, for being great friends.

My scientific mentors: Richard Palmiter, Luis de Lecea, Anne Brunet, Ellen Covey, and Chuck Drabek. Thank you so much for the opportunity to work in your labs and learn how to do great science. Thanks also to some great former teachers of mine who helped me grow as a writer and presenter: Susan McConnell at Stanford, I.Y. Hashimoto at Whitman College, and Kristen Allen-Bentsen and Tim Curtis at Inglemoor High School.

Thanks to Natalie Farra, Tracy Tufaga, and Maria Bernard at Elsevier for shepherding me through this second edition. Thank you especially for helping me to design the book and allowing me to have so much influence and oversight. I know that authors don't usually have this good fortune, and I feel lucky to work with you. Thanks also to Mica Haley and April Graham for seeing me through the first Edition.

Most of the beautiful photographs found throughout this book were taken and donated by my friends and family: Linn Blakeney, Patricia Bonnavion, Alison Carter, Don Carter, and Brie Cross. Thanks for letting me butcher your masterpieces in the name of science.

Acknowledgments

Finally, I thank the faculty, staff, and students at Williams College for their support, friendship, and collegiality. I'm humbled by my friends and colleagues at Williams, and I'm lucky to have the opportunity to not only work with such talented students, but to work with them so closely that over the years we have become friends and colleagues.

I'm really blessed to know so many amazing people.

Part 1

Using design principles to present science

1

Scientists as designers

As scientists, we don't normally think of ourselves as designers. If anything, we think of design in terms of designing the best scientific experiments. Yet when it comes to scientific presentations, all scientists should embrace design. If a scientific idea matters, then the design and delivery of a presentation necessary to communicate that idea matters. Fortunately, you don't need a special degree or certificate to think like a designer. You just need to care.

Designing Science Presentations. https://doi.org/10.1016/B978-0-12-815377-2.00001-9

The elements of a science presentation

The most important element in any science presentation is your scientific content: the ideas, experiments, and conclusions that you want to communicate with an audience. This book does not discuss methods of improving scientific content … that part is up to you. Indeed, this book is principally concerned with communicating your scientific content to an audience by designing a clear and effective presentation.

Other than your content, a science presentation consists of your story, your visual information, and your delivery.

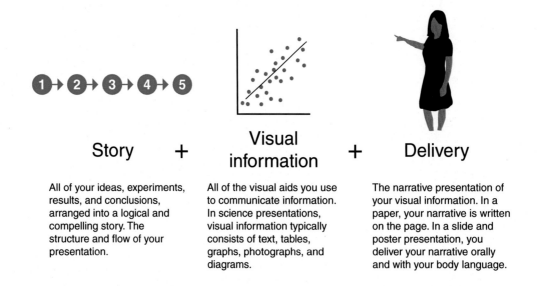

Story	+	Visual information	+	Delivery
All of your ideas, experiments, results, and conclusions, arranged into a logical and compelling story. The structure and flow of your presentation.		All of the visual aids you use to communicate information. In science presentations, visual information typically consists of text, tables, graphs, photographs, and diagrams.		The narrative presentation of your visual information. In a paper, your narrative is written on the page. In a slide and poster presentation, you deliver your narrative orally and with your body language.

To present your scientific content in the best possible way, much time and consideration should be devoted to optimizing your story, your visuals, and your delivery. And the best way to optimize these elements is through the process of design.

Good scientific content does not speak for itself

Experienced scientists know that good content does *not* speak for itself. When scientists fail to appreciate the importance of designing effective presentations, good studies are rejected by scientific journals, good ideas are denied by granting agencies, good stories are ignored by audiences, and good projects are passed by at poster sessions. Without a well-designed presentation, good science is essentially invisible.

The goal of designing a great presentation is not to take bad scientific content and disguise it as great. The goal is to communicate great content in a clear, succinct, and inspiring way … to value and respect your content by presenting it in the best possible light.

If you have spent time and effort pursuing a scientific goal, you owe it to yourself and your work to design and deliver a great presentation. Design matters because your content matters.

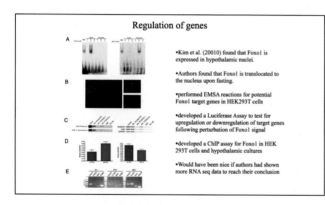

There may well be excellent scientific content on this slide, but it is highly inaccessible. The slide title does not convey a conclusion or take-home point. There are too many figures, each with seemingly different content. There is a lot of text, and its small size makes it hard to read. Any excellent science on this slide cannot speak for itself... it needs much better design to give it the attention it deserves.

Great design will not sell an inferior product, but it will enable a great product to achieve its maximum potential.

Thomas J. Watson Jr.
Design-focused former CEO of IBM

What is design?

Design is surprisingly hard to define. Most people think of design as the way something looks. While it is true that good design ultimately causes something to "look better," there is much more to design than just aesthetics.

Design is ultimately about determining what impact you want to have on an audience and then establishing the best way to achieve that objective.

One of the hallmarks of good design is that it is often invisible. The final product seems obvious, inevitable, and natural—like it could not have existed in any other way. In truth, well-designed science presentations indicate hard work on the part of the presenter, someone who intentionally chose what to add and what to take away to provide a deliberate experience to an audience.

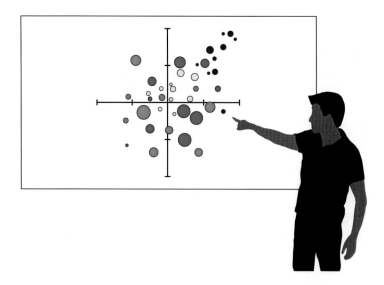

Good design is a lot like clear thinking made visual.

Edward Tufte
Data visualization and information design pioneer

Design is a plan for arranging elements in such a way as to accomplish a particular purpose.

Charles Eames
Designer and architect

What design is *not*

Design is not decoration. Design is not showing off the cute clip-art you found or the fancy tricks your presentation software can do. Design is not adding a random graphic to your poster or making text sparkle as it appears on a slide. Design is not adding anything meaningless that lacks information or purpose. Design is not anything that gets in the way.

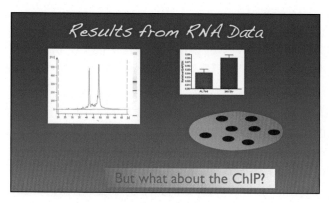

This slide is poorly designed, not because it is ugly (and many would consider it ugly!), but because it hasn't been designed to optimally communicate information with an audience. Instead of emphasizing the data and a larger conclusion, this slide emphasizes stylized font choices, distracting color patterns, and unnecessary clip art. This slide was *decorated* more than it was designed to communicate meaningful information.

Design does not call too much attention to itself. Design is not a way for scientists to show off how clever or brilliant they can be. Design is not about how many graphs can be placed on a slide, how many figures can be placed on a poster, or how many supplementary figures can be added to a research article.

Design is not accepting the default settings on presentation software, using pre-made templates, or blindly copying someone else's visual style without a purpose. Design is not laziness.

Design should never say, "Look at me."
It should always say, "Look at this."

David Craib
Visual communication designer

Design is not about what something looks like.
Design is about how it works.

Steve Jobs
Design-focused former CEO of Apple

Well-designed presentations translate complex information into a simple message

One of the key tenets of good design is striving for simplicity. To design a simple presentation means to distinguish between what is meaningful and what is unnecessary, focusing on the former and avoiding the latter. It is about filtering out all of the obvious, distracting, and unimportant elements in a presentation and focusing on what is truly important.

Simplicity doesn't tend to come naturally for us scientists. We are trained to think about and analyze complex datasets, keeping track of multiple details, numbers, and experiments throughout the day. How we process information in our own minds, however, is different from the best way to communicate this information to others.

The genius of a good presentation is often about what you leave out rather than what you put in. It is easy to add more and more facts, visual elements, and discussion to a presentation. It is much harder to subtract, deliberately taking away elements that don't add much value.

A simple presentation is not synonymous with a boring presentation. In fact, many of the most memorable, effective presentations are also the most focused. They resonate with audiences, sometimes long after they are presented, because everything in them is important and impactful.

Before

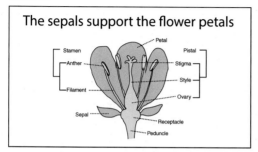

After

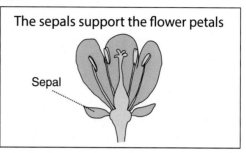

Increasing the simplicity of a presentation isn't the same as "dumming it down." It is about taking away unnecessary distractions or superfluous details so that the audience can focus on what is most important.

Simplicity is about subtracting the obvious and adding the meaningful.

John Maeda
Designer and technologist

A designer knows he has achieved perfection not when there is nothing left to add, but when there is nothing left to take away.

Antoine de Saint-Exupery
Writer and poet

Design is ultimately about the audience

What does it mean to design an effective presentation? Ultimately, the quality of a presentation is measured by its ability to impact an audience—the people reading your paper or grant proposal, or the people attending your talk or poster. Therefore, the best way to ensure that your presentation will succeed is to design a presentation not for you, but for the people who you want to impact.

Design is ultimately about the end user. Therefore, a well-designed science presentation must be made with the audience in mind.

You can design presentations for your audience in multiple ways:

- Determine who your audience will be and what they are likely to already know and not know. Design an introduction that quickly conveys necessary information while avoiding obvious background material.

- Consider the strengths and limitations of your presentation format. Design a presentation that plays to the strengths and, whenever possible, makes up for the limitations.

- Design tables, figures, diagrams, and photographs that quickly convey information to an audience.

- When appropriate, design strategies to emotionally engage your audience. Take advantage of presentation elements likely to appeal to emotion, enthusiasm, passion, or concern.

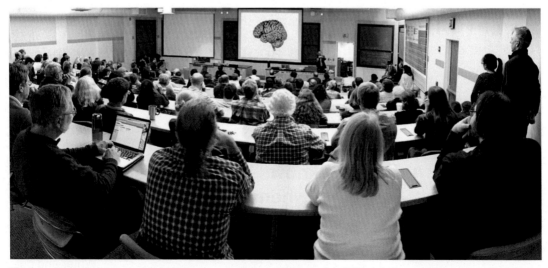

These people who have come to watch your presentation.... Who are they? What do they need to know so that they understand your science? Do they have preconceptions or biases about your topic? Are they likely to be tired? Hungry? What is necessary to hold their attention and explain topics with clarity?

Design is about more than just following "the rules"

The principles of good design can sometimes come across like a list of rules. This book is filled with many suggestions that might seem to limit freedom rather than inspire creativity. Interestingly, the opposite is true. These guidelines promote good design rather than limit it.

The rules of design are something like a dance routine. Without learning the right moves, you look like a fool on the dance floor. But once you know the proper steps, your freedom and creativity increases and you can express yourself in new and inventive ways.

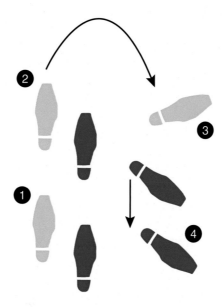

Also like dancing, it is occasionally okay to break a rule. Good dancers often break from prescribed dance moves, adding a stylistic flourish while keeping within their traditional routine. Likewise, it is sometimes beneficial to break from tradition and ignore a design guideline. The key is to be aware of *why* you are breaking a rule and what benefit it adds to your presentation.

Any scientist can learn to design excellent presentations

Some people are intimidated by the concept of presentation design because they "aren't designers." Indeed, the term "designer" seems to imply having an advanced skill set or attending some sort of professional design program. However, you don't need any special credentials to learn how to design a great presentation—design is really a *process*, a way of thinking about how to impact an audience.

All you need to do to practice design is to *choose* design as a process. By choosing to design, you choose to create the best possible experience for your audience. You reject lazy default presentation choices, old habits, dogma, and quick fixes for an active, deliberate approach.

Artistic tricks come with time and experience, but they are ultimately not what good design is all about. Good design is about determining how you want to impact an audience and then determining the best methods to achieve those goals.

Design is not the narrow application of formal skills, it is a way of thinking.

Christopher Pullman
Graphic designer

Appreciate good presentation design from other scientists

Thinking like a designer includes appreciating the design around you. Deliberately seek out great science presentations and identify what makes them so great. There is nothing like experiencing something outstanding to make you want to produce something similarly great. Likewise, there is nothing like experiencing a lackluster presentation to make you want to accomplish much more with your own work. Anyone in a scientific institution has access to numerous examples of papers, talks, and posters:

- Keep a file of research articles that are well written or that contain well-designed figures, regardless of their content.

- In your institution, learn who gives the best talks and always try to attend their presentations.

- At a poster session, spend time walking around the venue just to find and appreciate well-designed posters. If you are at an institution that has posters hanging around the hallways, walk around just to ask yourself which posters you like best.

- Watch a great science talk online. In an age of YouTube, iTunes University, and other online sites, there are literally thousands of amazing talks at your fingertips.

As Pablo Picasso famously said, "Good artists copy, great artists steal." Identify the design characteristics you see in outstanding science presentations and continually adopt them as your own.

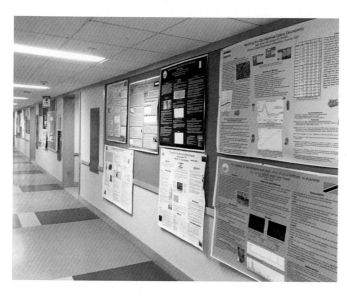

At most academic institutions, hallways are lined with old scientific posters from previous poster sessions. What a fantastic opportunity to take a walk and survey scientific presentation design. Ask yourself which posters stand out as being clear and accessible? What elements can you adopt as your own, and what irritating choices can you avoid?

Design is a continuous process

One of the most fun aspects about designing science presentations is that your attitude and vision continuously evolve. Not only do your abilities grow over time, you also start to see the same concept in different ways. For example, some scientists teach the same college course over many years. Each time the course is offered, they rediscover old presentation slides and realize that there is room for improvement, that the slides can be simpler and more effective, and that there are better and more efficient ways of communicating their messages to their students.

Design is like biological evolution—it never culminates in something that is finished or perfect, but the results are usually great for their time.

Obviously, at some point, you must decide that it is time to finish a presentation. Try not to be intimidated by deadlines, or let the perfect be the enemy of the good. An old saying at Apple, attributed to Steve Jobs, was that "Real Artists Ship," meaning that while it is important to make something as good as possible, it is even more important to finish a product and deliver it to users on time. Likewise, Real Scientists Publish. To succeed, scientists must regularly submit manuscripts and present their work.

Declaring something ready for publication or ready to be presented is not the same as declaring it perfect.

Each presentation is another evolution in your development as a designer, and another experience to learn from for the future.

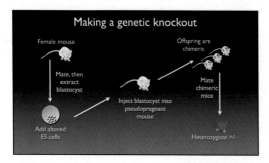 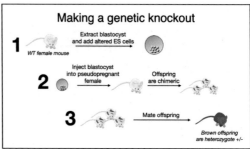

Evolution in the design process. These two slides were designed by the same instructor for the same molecular biology course, but the design on the left preceded the design on the right by four years.

Summary: Thinking like a designer

- Besides the content, a scientific presentation is composed of your story (sequence of information), your visual aids, and your delivery. Each can be optimized using principles of design to have a maximum impact on an audience.

- Good scientific content is not sufficient to impact an audience. Without a well-designed presentation, good science cannot speak for itself. Therefore, the purpose of designing a science presentation is to present good content in the best possible light.

- Design is the process of determining what impact you want to have on an audience and then determining the best way to accomplish that goal.

- Design is not about what something looks like, or about flashy, glittery visuals. Design is not about decorating—it is about achieving an end goal. Usually well-designed presentations turn out to be beautiful and visually appealing, but that is not the goal in itself.

- One of the hallmarks of good design is making the complex as simple as possible. Science is inherently complex, so determining ways to distill this complexity to an audience in an accessible manner is a challenge. Sometimes the genius of a good science presentation is what you choose to leave out rather than what you choose to include.

- Learning principles of design might seem like learning a list of rules, but these guidelines actually increase freedom and creativity. Like learning dance moves, design principles provide a framework for expressing yourself, a baseline from which you can add your own ideas and stylistic flourishes.

- Any scientist can learn to design excellent presentations. Good design skills don't require a formal skill set … good design is really a way of thinking.

- One way to increase design skills and a sense of taste is to appreciate the design around you. Keep a file of great scientific figures, attend great scientific talks, and survey great scientific posters at poster sessions. Observing great presentations is inspiring.

- Always remember that design is a continuous process. Declaring a presentation finished is not the same thing as declaring it perfect, and taste and style can mature over time. Have fun, and don't let the perfect be the enemy of the good.

2

Design goals for different presentation formats

The ways in which scientists share their work and ideas with others have changed dramatically over time, even in just the past 20 years. The ubiquity of fast, personal computers, in combination with easy-to-use software applications like Word, PowerPoint, Keynote, Photoshop, and Illustrator, have made any scientist capable of designing presentations in a variety of formats. In the modern scientific era, most scientists communicate via written presentations, oral presentations with slides, oral presentations without slides, and poster presentations. When designing a presentation from scratch, the first step is to consider the specific goals, strengths, and limitations of each presentation format to determine the best ways of communicating information.

Designing Science Presentations. https://doi.org/10.1016/B978-0-12-815377-2.00002-0

Each presentation format has unique goals

Every science presentation shares the ultimate goal of communicating information to an audience. However, each presentation format has additional goals that you can achieve if you design your presentation with that format in mind.

The written presentation

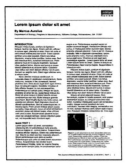

The goal of research or review articles is to permanently add detailed information or discussion to the scientific record. The goal of grants or fellowship proposals is to justify funding for a scientific project and convince the reader that you can accomplish your goals. Although it is possible to receive feedback on written presentations during the anonymous peer review process, these presentations are usually a one-way flow of information from author to reader.

Major categories of written presentations: primary research articles, review articles, grant/fellowship proposals.

The slide presentation

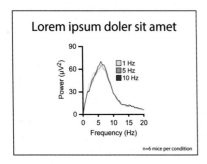

The goal of a slide presentation is to connect and communicate directly with your audience while using a series of powerful visual aids. Unlike other presentation formats, slides allow you to show anything you want, *whenever* you want. Depending on the format, two-way communication is often possible during the presentation or immediately following your talk.

Major categories of slide presentations: research seminars, symposium talks, lab meetings, journal clubs, data blitzes, course lectures.

The oral presentation (without slides)

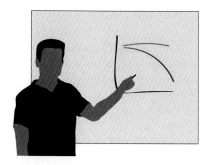

An oral presentation is an opportunity to present information without prepared visual aids. Although this format denies you a powerful visual tool, it also allows you to adjust your presentation in real-time depending on the questions and comments from your audience. The ultimate goal is to lead a conversation while demonstrating your mastery of the subject matter and your ability to think on your feet.

Major categories of oral presentations: chalk talks, round table presentations, elevator speeches, speaker introductions.

The poster presentation

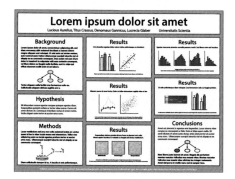

A scientific poster is a large visual document that allows you to quickly summarize (in about 5 min) a complete scientific project. The goal is to discuss science directly with other scientists, to solicit immediate feedback on your work, and to network with others.

Major categories of poster presentations: departmental/institutional poster sessions, scientific meeting poster sessions.

Advantages and disadvantages of different presentation formats

No presentation format is perfect. Each has its own implicit benefits and drawbacks that affect your ability to communicate science with an audience. Designing a good science presentation therefore requires an appreciation of these advantages and disadvantages, playing to the strengths of each format while making up for its limitations.

	Advantages	Disadvantages
Written	• The only format that is truly "published" • Considered a permanent entry into the scientific record • Reaches a global audience • Can present details of your methods and data • Editorial and review process can make a submitted manuscript much stronger	• You don't get to meet and network with your audience • No direct or immediate feedback on your work • Journal guidelines can limit your freedom • Difficult or impossible to convey emotion or enthusiasm • Peer reviewers can insert content or design choices with which you disagree
Slide	• Allows for emotion, enthusiasm, personality • More freedom to design with visual elements • Can use movies, animations, visual effects to enhance the meaning of data • Can interact with your audience and answer questions	• Not permanent or published • Only viewed by those present • Cannot go into detail about methods • Can cause presentation anxiety
Oral (without slides)	• Allows for emotion, enthusiasm, personality • Can interact with your audience and answer questions • Can adapt your presentation throughout depending on how your audience responds • No preparation of professional visuals is necessary	• Not permanent or published • Only viewed by those present • Cannot go into detail about methods • Cannot show photographs, animations, etc. • Can cause presentation anxiety
Poster	• Facilitates meeting and interacting with other scientists • Quickly communicates information • Conference/meeting attendees can provide immediate feedback	• Not permanent or published (but can be referenced) • Only viewed by conference/meeting attendees • Cannot present a large volume of information • Hard to show movies/sounds without accessory devices

Reasons for success and failure

Science presentations can succeed or fail to communicate or resonate with audiences regardless of their scientific content. Although content certainly matters, the composition, visual design, and delivery of your presentation are what will ultimately make your presentation a success.

Different categories of presentations succeed or fail for different reasons. When designing a presentation for a specific format, be mindful about the best ways to succeed in that format. At the same time, be cautious about common pitfalls that might cause a failure to communicate with your audience.

	Reasons for success	Reasons for failure
Written	• The writing is clear and articulate • Excellent transitions provide a steady narrative and a natural flow of information to the reader • Detailed figures and tables stand on their own but are well-integrated into the text	• Poor writing prevents the reader from understanding the message • Poor flow of information causes the paper to seem jumbled and without direction • A lack of rationale or motivation makes the content seem trivial or unimportant • Typos and grammatical errors cause annoying distractions and suggest incompetence
Slide	• Visual information complements oral delivery so that the audience clearly understands the message • Visual information instantly conveys data and concepts to the audience • The talk is easy to follow • The subject matter comes across as important and interesting • The audience perceives the enthusiasm and excitement of the speaker	• No sense of goal or purpose • No sense of narrative or story • Slides are poorly designed • Slides distract from the main message • Poor oral delivery • Too many words or figures per slide • No consideration for the needs of the audience • No enthusiasm in the speaker
Oral (without slides)	• Presenter dynamically conveys information and interest through verbal delivery and body language • The personality of the speaker enhances the message • Audience perceives a clear message	• The presenter is unable to communicate without visual aids • The presenter fails to engage the audience
Poster	• The presenter fosters discussion and solicits feedback • Visual information complements concise text • Oral presentation to visitors is succinct and informative	• Too much text • Too many figures that take too much time to comprehend • Awkward presentation of poster with visitors (or complete absence of the presenter) during poster session • No solicitation of discussion or feedback

Summary: Designing for different presentation formats

- Science presentations typically take the form of a written publication, a slide presentation, an oral presentation without slides, or a poster presentation. Each presentation has specific advantages and disadvantages, as well as different reasons for success or failure in communicating with an audience.

- Design a science presentation while cognizant of the specific advantages and disadvantages of your presentation format. Design a presentation while playing to the strengths of your format while doing your best to make up for the limitations.

- Don't assume that your presentation will automatically be a success because you have great scientific content. Be cognizant of the best ways to communicate in each presentation format while avoiding common pitfalls that can afflict other presenters.

- Don't design a science presentation for one format as you would for another ... be mindful of the design considerations for each.

Part 2

Visual elements in science presentations

3

Color

Color is a powerful communication tool. It can group information into categories and show meaningful relationships between data. It can seize an audience's attention and direct people's eyes to a specific point in space. It can also create a mood or tone that evokes emotions and attitudes. Poorly chosen colors distract from your presentation and can make your content unreadable. In contrast, well-chosen colors help illuminate and emphasize your message while making your presentation more compelling and memorable.

Designing Science Presentations. https://doi.org/10.1016/B978-0-12-815377-2.00003-2

Use color to communicate

Presentation applications like PowerPoint and Keynote make it easy to select from millions of colors for text, graphics, backgrounds, foregrounds, etc. Adding color is a great way to add liveliness and visual energy to a presentation … however, it is most powerful when it has a purpose. Like all other visual elements, color should be used for design, not for decoration.

We should use color to better communicate with our audiences. Color is a wonderful tool to highlight information, to enhance a message, or to convey an atmosphere or emotion.

When a scientist chooses colors poorly, the message conveyed in a figure, slide, or poster can be obscured. At worst, presentations become unreadable. However, good decisions about color can make the main points of a presentation memorable. Color can emphasize specific data, highlight specific conclusions, and convey messages to audiences faster than words alone. Color can also create a striking visual aesthetic that enhances the tone of your presentation and conveys emotion to an audience.

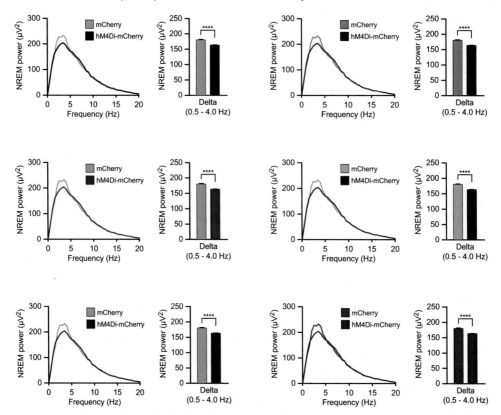

When presenting scientific information, there are lots of possible color choices and combinations. Instead of choosing colors randomly, deliberately make choices that are designed to emphasize the main message. Are some colors most intuitively paired with certain datasets? What information is most interesting and should appear in the foreground? What information is best in the background?

When scientists use color to decorate rather than to design, their slides and posters can look like a trip to the circus. A misconception is that lots of color will excite audiences or create a playful atmosphere. In reality, poor color choices are distracting, overwhelming, and sometimes indecipherable.

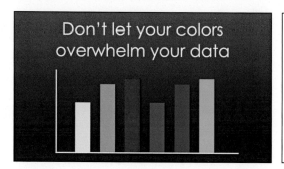
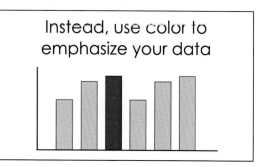

How to describe color

Most computer applications assume that you already know the vocabulary of color, even though few people understand all of these terms. Understanding the vocabulary of color will help you make informed decisions when choosing colors for your presentations.

Hue is a color's purest identity, independent of other values such as lightness, darkness, and saturation. Hues are what come to mind when you think of a color in its purest, most fundamental form.

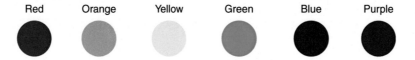

The **primary colors**, red, yellow, and blue, are the three colors that cannot be created by mixing any other colors.

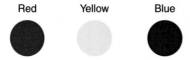

Secondary colors results from the mixing of two of the primary colors.

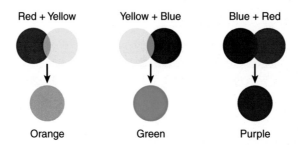

Intermediate colors result from mixing a primary and secondary color, or multiple secondary colors.

Shade is the amount of black added to a hue.

Tint is the amount of white added to a hue.

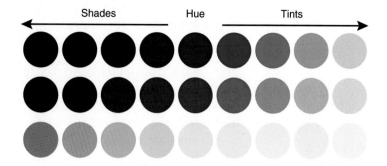

Value (or **intensity**) refers to the inherent lightness or darkness of a color. The value of different colors can be compared relative to a black-and-white gradient. Black has the highest value and white has the lowest value. The values of colors become important when choosing color combinations that contrast well with each other.

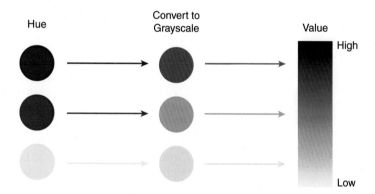

Saturation refers to the degree of hue in a color. A fully saturated color is a true hue, while colors with less saturation look more and more gray. When you convert colors to grayscale, the colors are completely de-saturated.

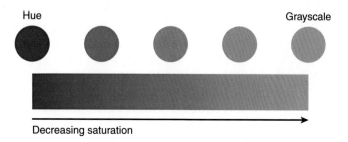

How computers specify color

Computers specify color in different formats. The optimal format to choose depends on whether your presentation will be printed (e.g., papers, handouts, and posters) or displayed digitally (e.g., slide presentations and web documents).

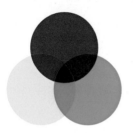

CMYK

The CMYK format is used to specify color for printed documents. Color printers use a combination of cyan (C), magenta (M), yellow (Y), and black (K) inks to produce all hues of the color spectrum. Each hue is specified as combinations of each ink source. A particular color is specified by a value for C, M, Y, and K ranging from 0 to 100. Use this color specification system for written and poster presentations so that your presentation will be consistent from printer to printer.

Red = CMYK (0,100,100,0)

Blue = CMYK (100,100,0,0)

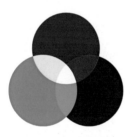

RGB

The RGB format is used to specify how color will appear on computer displays, television screens, and digital projectors. Each pixel is composed of a combination of red (R), green (G), and blue (B) hues. When all three hues are combined equally, the result is white light. A particular color is specified by a value for R, G, and B, each with a range of 0–255. Use this color specification system for slide presentations.

Red = RGB (255,0,0)

Blue = RGB (0,0,255)

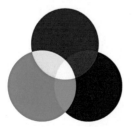

Hexvalue

Website colors also use combinations of red, green, and blue, but utilize a six-digit number instead of the RGB specification system. Colors are specified in the format "#RRGGBB" in which RR, GG, and BB are the values for the red, green, and blue values of each color, respectively. The degree of each color ranges from #00 to #FF. This color specification system is used when designing websites.

Red = ##(FF0000)

Blue = ##(0000FF)

A color wheel can be helpful in selecting colors

A color wheel depicts the full color spectrum and helps show how different colors relate to each other. The three primary hues (red, yellow, and blue) are spaced evenly apart. Secondary and intermediate colors are spaced in between the primary colors. The center of the wheel has increasing tints while the outside of the wheel has increasing shades.

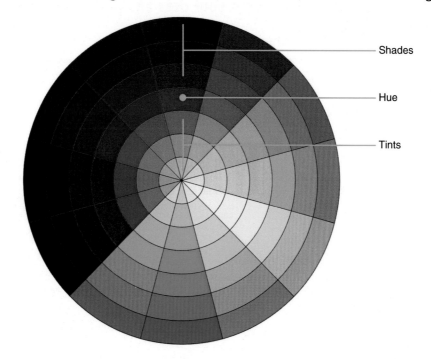

Presentation applications feature their own versions of color wheels, but the overall concept of a color wheel is always the same: to depict relationships between different hues.

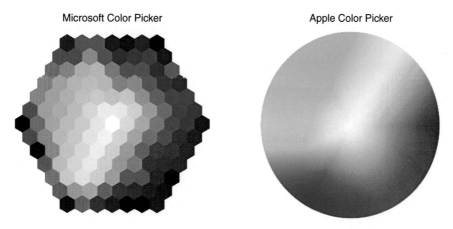

Microsoft Color Picker

Apple Color Picker

Choosing color combinations using a color wheel

When you need to use multiple colors for graphs or diagrams, a color wheel can help you choose combinations that visually emphasize differences between different datasets.

Different combinations of monochromatic, complementary, or analogous colors will convey different meanings about your data and presentation themes.

Monochromatic

Only one hue in various shades or tints. The advantage to this strategy is that it creates a consistent, unified look. Even though different datasets may be categorized differently (e.g., different bars on a bar graph), they seem representative of a larger, uniform category.

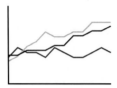 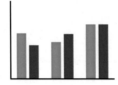 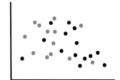

Complementary

Two or three hues on opposite sides of a color wheel. This strategy enhances the difference between categories of data and makes them seem more like opposites.

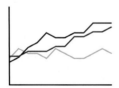 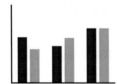 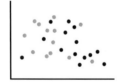

Analogous

Two or three hues that are relatively adjacent on the color wheel. This strategy combines elements of both the monochromatic and complementary strategies, using multiple colors while also achieving a consistent, harmonious look.

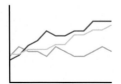 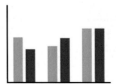 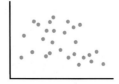

Monochromatic

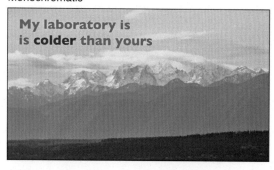

Complementary

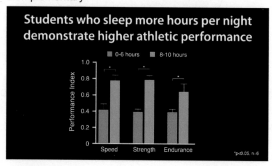

Analogous

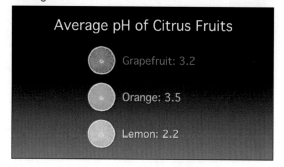

The colors that you choose to represent your data
and ideas will affect the tone of your presentation and
how your audience perceives relationships.

Choose warm colors for the foreground

Colors on opposite sides of the color wheel are often described as "warm" or "cool." Warm colors consist of pinks, reds, oranges, and yellows, and are associated with energy, vitality, excitement, and fun. Cool colors are made up of greens, blues, and purples, and are associated with peace, serenity, and nature.

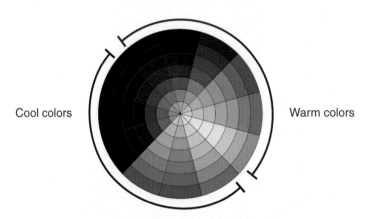

Cool colors   Warm colors

Humans are hard-wired to attend to warm colors more than cool colors. Furthermore, we perceive warm colors as being in the foreground and cool colors as being in the background. Therefore, choose warm colors to highlight the data that you really want to emphasize.

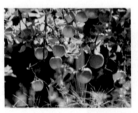

People are hard-wired to focus their attention on warm colors, such as reds, oranges, and yellows. This phenomenon is no doubt a consequence of human evolution, as salient environmental stimuli like fruits, animals, and potentially harmful stimuli are often composed of warm colors, while cooler blues, greens, and browns typically make up the background.

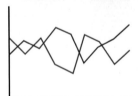

The red line appears in the foreground even though it is technically placed behind the blue line

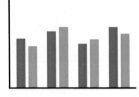

The orange bars attract attention much more than the blue bars

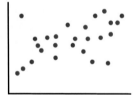

The red data points stand out even though the green data points show more of a trend

Ensure foreground and background colors have high contrast

In written presentations, backgrounds are almost always white. In slide and poster presentations, you have more freedom to choose different colors for background and foreground combinations. Considerations for choosing colors in each kind of presentation format are described in other chapters, however, no matter which format you use, you must choose background and foreground colors with optimal contrast. Ideally, the colors you choose for your foreground and background should be as far apart in value as possible to maximize visibility.

The best foreground and background combinations are black on a white background or white on a black background. If using color, a warm color foreground usually stands out on a darker cool color background.

To test various foreground/background combinations, convert your colors to grayscale. Red and green colors are terrible together because they are so close in value. Yellow and blue combinations are better together because they are relatively far apart in value. Because yellow is a warm color, it looks better on a blue background than blue will look on a yellow background. The more your two colors approach the colors of black and white, the greater the contrast and the easier your visuals will be to perceive.

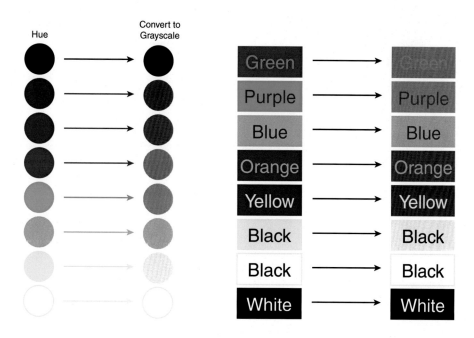

Use color to highlight salient information

Warm colors are excellent for highlighting data in any kind of figure. For color to be effective in attracting an audience's attention, it should ideally be used in isolation.

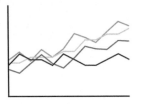
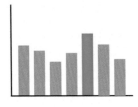
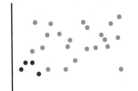

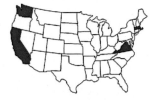
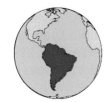

	X	Y	Z
A	15.4	12.3	11.1
B	14.8	15.8	19.9
C	10.4	10.6	14.7
D	10.9	41.2	14.1
E	14.2	16.3	12.1

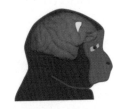

ATTTGACGATGAGCGCTAGCATGGACCGAT
TAAACTGCTACTCGCGATCGTACCTGGCTA

Emotional associations of different colors

Hues are not emotionally neutral. Because of our cultural experiences and the colors of items found in nature, each hue can express a different personality. Choose colors with an appreciation for these emotional associations, as they can affect an audience's attitude, even unconsciously. The colors that you choose for foreground and background, and even the colors that you wear, can all affect your audience's mood.

 **White:** purity, simplicity, innocence, clean, spacious, milk, cotton, clouds

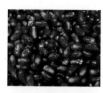 **Red:** love, hate, passion, hot, stop signal, blood, berries, heart

 **Yellow:** light, cheerful, sunny, optimistic, summer, dry, wheatfield, cornfield

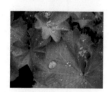 **Green:** natural, environment, healthy, go signal, grass, vegetables, trees

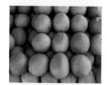 **Orange:** autumn, fruity, fun, sporty, pumpkin, Halloween, caution sign, oranges

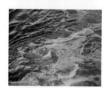 **Blue:** peaceful, natural, tranquil, calm, positive, melancholy, cold, sky, air, water, ocean, ice

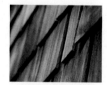 **Brown:** rustic, earthy, woody, cozy, dirt, wilderness, cabin, outdoors

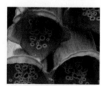 **Purple:** exotic, creative, sweet, artistic, flowers, candy

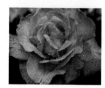 **Pink:** soft, delicate, young, sweet, feminine, flowers, baby, candy

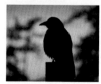 **Black:** powerful, formal, corporate, classy, night, suit, briefcase, judge

Prepare for color in a colorless environment

It is important to consider that approximately 10% of men and 1% of women have some form of color vision deficiency. In addition, many people print documents in black and white instead of color to save money on relatively expensive color ink cartridges. Therefore, it is wise to consider how your color choices will be perceived in black and white conditions.

Fortunately, even if someone isn't able to distinguish among different hues, anyone should be able to distinguish among differences in color value. No matter which colors you choose, test your color combinations in grayscale to ensure maximum contrast for audiences unable to perceive color.

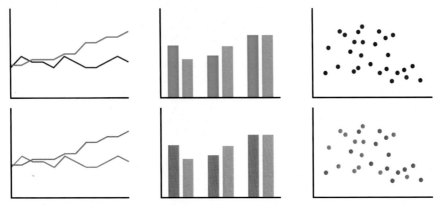

To see how your data will be perceived in a black and white environment, convert your colors to grayscale. Colors that are close in value, like red and green, become indistinguishable.

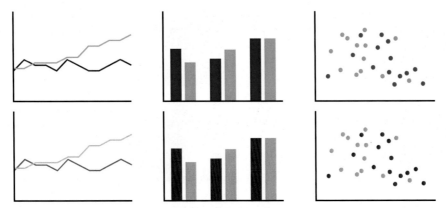

To make your data accessible in a colorless environment, choose colors that are far apart in value. If you want to use two colors that are close in value (for example, you want to use red and green because you are comparing red and green tomatoes), try using a tint of one color and a shade of the other to increase the contrast.

Black and white are colors, too

Don't ignore black, white, and shades of gray when choosing colors for a presentation. In written presentations, color figures can be unnecessary. Some journals charge high fees for color figures that could easily be made in black and white. Well-chosen shades of gray can be used in place of multiple colors.

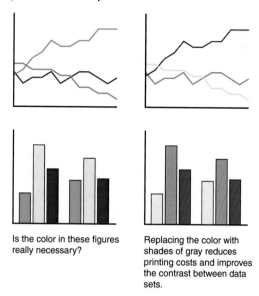

Is the color in these figures really necessary?

Replacing the color with shades of gray reduces printing costs and improves the contrast between data sets.

Even when there is no cost to using color, black and white can convey a strong, emotional tone. White and light grays convey a sense of purity and simplicity, while black and dark grays can convey strength, power, and professionalism.

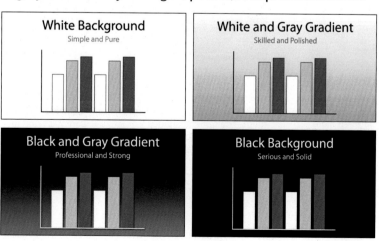

What you see on your screen might not be what you get

Science presentations are designed on a computer, where all visual elements are backlit by the computer screen. Printed documents and slides projected onto a screen are not backlit, so visual elements, especially colors, are likely to appear slightly differently.

To guarantee that your audience will see your figures and slides as you prepared them, preview them in their final form before presenting them to others. Otherwise, you might be surprised that your blues turn into purples, your reds turn into browns, and your yellows disappear altogether!

Always try printing figures and drafts of posters on a color printer before submitting a manuscript or printing a poster on large paper. Unless your color printer isn't functioning well, the final product is most likely to resemble what you printed versus what you see on your screen. Additionally, many poster printing centers (institutional printing centers or commercial printers like FedEx Office or Staples) will print a smaller preview of a poster before printing the correct size. Always examine these test versions to ensure that colors are represented as you intended.

For a slide presentation, try presenting some test slides in the presentation room before your presentation begins. Modern laptops have projector calibration settings integrated into their operating systems. If you don't know how to open and adjust these settings, it is worth the brief amount of time it will take to learn.

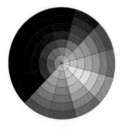

The beautiful color wheel that appears throughout this chapter. On a glossy computer display, the colors appear even more brilliant than they do in print.

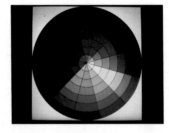

A photograph of the color wheel when digitally projected onto a white screen in a dark seminar room. The darkest shades appear almost black and some of the inner tints are too white.

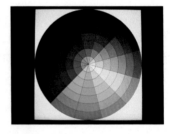

A photograph of the same digitally projected wheel after adjusting the settings on both the computer and projector.

Summary: Design principles for color

- Color is a great tool to enhance communication in papers, slides, and posters. Color is most effective when it is used deliberately to highlight information, not when it is used to decorate.

- There are some simple ways of describing color. Hues represent colors in their purest form. Increasing the tint or shade of a hue makes that hue lighter or darker, respectively. The value of a color is how light/dark it appears in grayscale. Decreasing the saturation of a hue removes its color value and brings it closer to grayscale.

- Computers specify color in different formats: CMYK, RGB, and Hexvalue. CMYK is best for printed documents (papers and posters), RGB is best for slides, and Hexvalue is used in website design.

- A color wheel is helpful to visualize the relationships between different colors. Different color combinations of monochromatic, complementary, or analogous colors on a color wheel will convey different meanings about your data.

- Warm colors (pinks, reds, oranges, and yellows) naturally appear in the foreground. Cool colors (greens, blues, and purples) naturally appear in the background.

- Ensure that foreground and background colors have high contrast in color value. If you convert your color combinations to grayscale, you can better visualize the contrast in value.

- Color is a wonderful tool to highlight information. For color to be effective as a highlighter, it should be used sparsely.

- Different colors have different emotional associations based on past experiences. It is worth considering these associations when choosing colors for datasets, diagrams, and foreground/background colors.

- To ensure that colorblind individuals will be able to read color figures and slides (as well as people who print your documents on a black and white printer), choose color combinations that differ in color value. That way anyone should be able to distinguish between two or more colors, even if they cannot perceive the saturation of those colors.

- Remember that black and white are perfectly fine color choices for presentations, and blacks, whites, and shades of gray can also convey emotion to an audience.

- After preparing figures or slides, always preview how they will look in print or when projected to ensure the final version is consistent with what you see on your computer screen.

4

Typography

Typography is the art of selecting and arranging characters to make language visible. It is hard to remember that before the 1980s, most people werre limited to using one or two fonts on typewriters for all of their decisions about type. After the debut of the first Apple MacIntosh, anyone could select from dozens of fonts, each with their own characteristics and personality, and make decisions about font size, line spacing, and alignment. The design decisions we make about type have consequences for the legibility of text, the clarity of our main points, and even the meanings of words themselves.

Designing Science Presentations. https://doi.org/10.1016/B978-0-12-815377-2.00004-4

Decisions about text matter

We see text so often in our everyday lives that we forget that every use of text and typography involves choices: choices about font, character size, casing, typesetting, etc. Decisions about typography matter because they affect the legibility, meaning, and tone of the language we use.

Just as you can speak the same word in many different ways, the way you write a word can convey emotion and attitude in addition to the meaning of the word itself.

Before   After

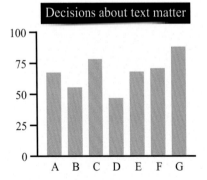
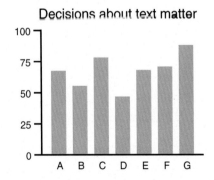

Characteristics of a font

What are the attributes of a font that confer its personality? Fonts are commonly classified as having serifs (slight projections finishing off a stroke of a letter) or not having serifs (called a sans serif font).

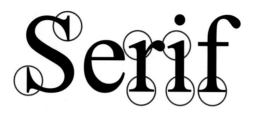

Besides the presence or absence of serifs, each font has its own height (distance from baseline to cap height), weight (thickness of lines), and counters (shape of the negative space within letters).

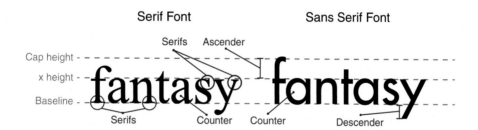

Notice how different the word "fantasy" appears in these two different fonts. The serif font (Times New Roman) has a smaller cap height and line width than the sans serif font (Futura). Also notice the difference in counters in the letter "a."

Choose the right font for the job

Fonts convey tone and personality. Knowing which font to use in a presentation depends on the attitude you wish to convey, as well as which will be most legible in your presentation format.

Serif fonts are good for smaller character sizes (10–14 pts) in multiple lines of type. The serifs guide the letters into one another so it is easier for the reader to follow one line at a time. Most books and magazines are written in a serif font. (This book is an exception because most of the page space is taken up by figures, in which sans serif fonts are optimal). In general, manuscripts are best written in serif fonts.

Font	Personality
Garamond	classic, refined
Georgia	elegant, mature
Times New Roman	professional, traditional

Sans serif fonts are usually perceived as most simple and pure, as they lack stylistic serifs or flourish. They are easier to see and perceive from a distance, as in billboards or theater marquees. These fonts are therefore best for slide and poster presentations in which an audience must be able to read text from across a room.

Font	Personality
Calibri	formal, neutral
Century Gothic	grand, optimistic
Helvetica	simple, pure, contemporary

Some sans serif fonts convey a bit more personality than others. They are more playful and can make a presentation seem less standard or routine.

Font	Personality
Futura	fun, utopia
Gill Sans	warm, friendly
Myriad Pro	jovial, friendly, casual

Some sans serif fonts are extremely playful. They are typically chosen because they add an informal, jovial tone to a presentation. However, this can also be a problem. These fonts may be conspicuously playful in a way that draws attention from the main message. They may also make a presenter come across as trying too hard to be fun. Give these fonts good consideration before using them, and consider using a slightly more professional font such as Gill Sans or Myriad Pro.

Font	Personality
Chalkboard	informal, fun
Comic Sans	silly, fun
Marker Felt	informal, creative

Non-proportional (also called "monospaced") fonts are fonts in which each character has the same width. This is in contrast to most fonts, in which letters like "m" and "w" have larger widths than "i" or "l." Non-proportional typefaces were originally designed for typewriters, which could only move the same distance for any letter typed. Nowadays they are great for writing letters in a sequence, such as sequences of DNA, amino acids, or computer code.

Font	Personality
Courier	retro, nerdy
Letter Gothic	simple, elementary
Lucida Sans Typewriter	informal, quirky

Specialty fonts convey a lot of personality and tone. They are ideal during moments when you want to conspicuously capture an audience's attention and convey an attitude. They can easily overshadow the message of a presentation, therefore they are best used in isolation, such as in title slides, flyers, or when emphasizing a major take-home point. These fonts are usually illegible at small sizes and look best in sizes 30 pts and above.

ADVENTURE

PRINCETOWN LET

The New Yorker

Considerations for casing

Casing refers to the degree to which you use capitalized letters. In an **ALL-UPPERCASE** format, every single letter is capitalized. This format adds emphasis and weight to a title, but can be difficult to read unless the letters are very large. In **Title Case** format, all words are capitalized except for certain subsets of words such as articles, prepositions, conjunctions, and forms of "to be." This format is used most often for titles, such as the titles of books and movies. In **Sentence case** format, only the first letter of the first word is capitalized, along with proper nouns. This format is how most text is written (sentences you find in papers, books, magazines, etc.). Finally, in an **all-lowercase** format, no capitalization is used.

```
 UPPERCASE   I LIKE TO EAT CHOCOLATES AT BURROW'S CAFE

Title Case   I Like to Eat Chocolates at Burrow's Cafe

Sentence case   I like to eat chocolates at Burrow's Cafe

 lowercase   i like to eat chocolates at burrow's cafe
```

Considerations for different casing styles in various presentation media are described throughout this book, but certain guidelines apply. In general, it is usually best to avoid the all-uppercase format unless you use few words and the letters are very large (for example, subheadings on a poster). Title case is best for major heading titles, while sentence case is best for the titles of subsections of a written document or poster, and the titles of figures or figure legends.

Sometimes, a scientific word needs to be in all-uppercase letters. If the word is long, it can often visually overpower a sentence. In these circumstances, try reducing the font size of the uppercase word by 1–2 pts to make the sentence appear more balanced.

We characterized the role of CMTRPB-3 in cognitive enhancement.

We characterized the role of CMTRPB-3 in cognitive enhancement.

In the top sentence, the name of the compound in all caps, CMTRPB-3, is large and seems to overpower the sentence. In the bottom sentence, the name is reduced in size by two pts. relative to the other words and the sentence seems more balanced.

Choose font styles to increase legibility

Each decision you make about type, including casing (uppercase vs. lowercase), style (bold, italics, etc.), size, underlining, and color, will affect the legibility of your sentences.

When designing a presentation, it can be fun to experiment with the available options for fonts, but unless you have good reason to make an exception, your end goal should be to choose text that is the most legible.

In general, don't use all caps. Use italics to emphasize a specific word but not to stylize an entire sentence. Some fonts are easier to read in bold—test your font of choice to see what is most legible. Don't choose colors that are hard to see. Similarly, don't write sentences in highly ornate fonts that are hard to read.

Easier to read

Some sentences are more legible than others.

Some sentences are more legible than others.

SOME SENTENCES ARE MORE LEGIBLE THAN OTHERS.

SOME SENTENCES ARE MORE LEGIBLE THAN OTHERS.

Some sentences are more legible than others.

Some sentences are more legible than others.

<u>Some sentences are more legible than others.</u>

SOME SENTENCES ARE MORE LEGIBLE THAN OTHERS.

SOME SENTENCES ARE MORE LEGIBLE THAN OTHERS.

<u>SOME SENTENCES ARE MORE LEGIBLE THAN OTHERS.</u>

Some sentences are more legible than others.

Some sentences are more legible than others.

Some sentences are more legible than others.

Some sentences are more legible than others.

Some sentences are more legible than others.

Some sentences are more legible than others.

Harder to read

Font considerations for numbers

When choosing fonts, be mindful about how your numbers appear. For example, the number one looks like an obvious 1 in some fonts, while in others it can look like the letter l.

Calibri	Century Gothic	Comic Sans	Courier	Garamond	Georgia	Gill Sans	Helvetica	Myriad Pro	Times New Roman
0	0	0	0	0	0	0	0	0	0
1	1	1	1	1	1	l	1	1	1
2	2	2	2	2	2	2	2	2	2
3	3	3	3	3	3	3	3	3	3
4	4	4	4	4	4	4	4	4	4
5	5	5	5	5	5	5	5	5	5
6	6	6	6	6	6	6	6	6	6
7	7	7	7	7	7	7	7	7	7
8	8	8	8	8	8	8	8	8	8
9	9	9	9	9	9	9	9	9	9

In figures, numbers in sans serif fonts are always the most legible. When in doubt, use Helvetica. It's always a good choice.

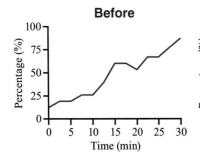

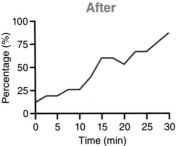

The graph on the left uses a serif font (Times New Roman). Almost all scientific journals suggest making figures in a sans serif font, such as the graph on the right (Helvetica), because these fonts are easier to read.

Make sure that superscript or subscript numbers are legible. Sometimes, depending on the font, it is optimal to change the font size of superscript or subscript characters so that the numbers become easier to read.

Before

$$1 \times 10^4 = 10^2 \times 10^2$$

After

$$1 \times 10^4 = 10^2 \times 10^2$$

The equation on the left was written using the default Helvetica settings in Microsoft Word. In the equation on the right, the superscript numbers are a bit more legible because the font size was increased by 1 pt. and the superscript settings were changed to raise the numbers by 1 pt.

Sizing up a font

A common misconception is that the size of a font is the distance from the bottom to the top of a character. In reality, a font size is the height of an imaginary metal block as would exist in an old-fashioned typewriter. Even in the modern computer era, a font size is the height of the assumed equivalent of the block.

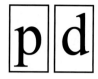

Computers specify the size of a font in "points." A point is defined as one-twelfth of a pica, which itself is about one-sixth of an inch.

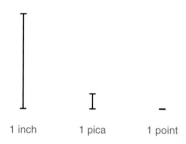

1 inch   1 pica   1 point

Because the point size is the height of an imaginary block in an old-fashioned typewriter and not the height of the character itself, the only way to know exactly how large a font will appear in a particular point size is to try it!

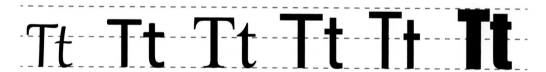

All of these letters are written in the same font size. The fonts, from left to right, are Gabriola, Calibri, Times New Roman, Helvetica, Futura, and Impact.

Making the best use of bullets

Bullets are a great way to group items into a list or sequence. Like any other visual element, their use should incorporate some simple design principles to increase clarity and communication.

Before	After	
Never use a single bullet • Bullets are for lists	**Never use a single bullet** Bullets are for lists	**Never use a single bullet.** Bullets are for lists. If you are only going to list one bullet item, just group it with the rest of the text.
Don't write wordy bullet items • The problem with writing long bullet items is that the eye has a difficult time reading several lines of text for a single bullet. • Even for written presentations, it is best to limit text to 1-3 lines. Otherwise, you are writing a paragraph!	Don't write wordy bullet items • Several lines of text are hard for the eye to read • Try to limit yourself to 1-2 lines instead of writing a paragraph	**Don't write wordy bullet items.** The eye has a hard time following bullets after about 3 lines.
Increase the spacing • Without good spacing, bulleted items are too close together • Without good spacing, bulleted items are too close together • Without good spacing, bulleted items are too close together	**Increase the spacing** • Without good spacing, bulleted items are too close together • Without good spacing, bulleted items are too close together • Without good spacing, bulleted items are too close together	**Increase the line space between bulleted items.** This spacing helps the audience visualize the separation between different bullet items.
Indent the text •Help your audience see bullets easier by indenting your text •Help your audience see bullets easier by indenting your text •Help your audience see bullets easier by indenting your text	Indent the text • Help your audience see bullets easier by indenting your text • Help your audience see bullets easier by indenting your text • Help your audience see bullets easier by indenting your text	**Indent the text on your bullets.** These indentations not only make your list look polished and professional but also help the audience differentiate between different bullet items.

Use numbers when you want to show a sequence and a symbol when the sequence is arbitrary.

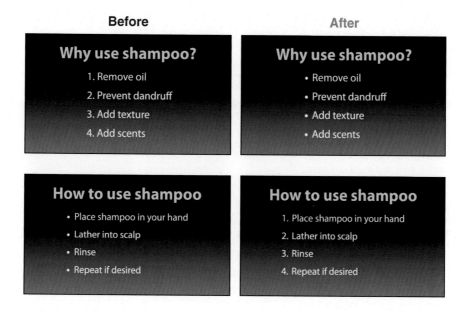

Use strategies to optimize clarity and legibility when using bullets:

- Keep your bullet list brief. Try not to include more than four to six items.

- Try starting each bullet item with an active verb.

- Be consistent throughout your entire bullet list in the verb tense that you use (past, present, or future; active or passive).

- Be consistent about whether your bullets end with punctuation.

- Keep your bullet style simple. Dots are much easier to perceive than alternatives.

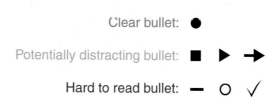

Be deliberate about typesetting

Typesetting refers to how characters are arranged together in a word, in a sentence, or on a page. Most people never consider changing the typesetting defaults on their computers, but sometimes changing the way words or blocks of text appear can have a powerful influence on the tone of a presentation, especially in slide presentations.

	Before	After
Varying the tracking (spacing) between characters can enhance the meaning of a word. Increasing the tracking makes words seem lighter and spacious; decreasing the tracking makes words seem tighter and more compact.	ATMOSPHERE	ATMOSPHERE
Changing the font height or size for specific words can enhance the meaning of those words. You can often convey the emotion of a word by literally changing how tall or big (or short and small) it appears.	SHORT AND TALL BIG AND SMALL	SHORT AND TALL BIG AND SMALL
Leading (pronounced "led-ing") is the spacing between lines of text. Some fonts naturally have a default leading that can seem too high or low. Adjust the leading for your font of choice so your text is perfectly spaced out.	Sometimes the leading is too high Sometimes the leading is too low	Sometimes the leading is just right
Try to avoid isolated words. Sometimes a single word at the end of a sentence can seem to exist in isolation by itself. Try resizing your lines so that no words are left alone by themselves.	It's never nice to have an isolated word	It's never nice to have an isolated word
Typeset blocks of text so they form solid shapes. Arranging text into block-like shapes makes your text seem more tightly organized and easier to read compared to the random shapes that can form due to the lengths of words that fit on different lines.	Sometimes the text you use forms an awkward two-dimensional shape on the page	Sometimes the text you use forms an awkward two-dimensional shape on the page

Summary: Design principles for typography

- As scientists, we don't usually think about choices about typography. However, decisions about text matter. They affect the legibility, meaning, and tone of the language we use.

- Most fonts are categorized as serif fonts or sans serif fonts. Serif fonts are especially good for written manuscripts and documents. Sans serif fonts are especially good for slide and poster presentations.

- Different font choices convey personality. Choose a font based on its legibility and also what sense of formality, seriousness, and fun you want to convey. Be careful not to choose an overly conspicuous font, such as Comic sans, that may distract from the content of your presentation.

- A simple, sans serif font, such as Helvetica, is best for text in figures.

- Non-proportional fonts, in which each character has the same width, are optimal for sequences of data, such as sequences of DNA, amino acids, or computer code.

- In general, most text in a presentation should be written in sentence case format, in which only the first letter of the first word is capitalized, along with proper nouns. Rarely use title case, in which all words are capitalized, because this form of casing is a bit harder to read. All-uppercase is especially hard to read for long phrases or sentences.

- Use italics or underlining to emphasize a specific word or phrase—emphasizing entire sentences in italics or underlining only make them harder to read.

- Consider how your font choices will affect the appearance of numbers, which are also displayed with the characteristics of your font's personality.

- Font sizes are hard to compare between fonts. Two fonts written in the same font size may not actually be the same size. The only way to know how large a font will appear in a particular point size is to try it!

- Use bullets to highlight items in a list or numbers to highlight sequences of information. Ensure that bulleted/numbered lists are optimized to quickly and concisely communicate information.

- Especially in slide presentations (but also in poster presentations and figures), consider how changing typesetting features will affect the look and legibility of your text. These typesetting decisions include the tracking (spacing) between characters in words, the font height and width, and the leading (the spacing between lines of text). Also consider how blocks of text appear on a slide, trying to avoid isolated words or awkward two-dimensional shapes of text.

5

Words

It is often possible to express the same idea using many different combinations of words and phrases. The English language is rich in vocabulary, and many words have similar meanings. The key to good writing is to select the best possible combination of words so that you can express your ideas as precisely, concisely, and clearly as possible.

Designing Science Presentations. https://doi.org/10.1016/B978-0-12-815377-2.00005-6

Word choice matters

All too often, scientists designing presentations think of what they want to say and then choose the first words that come to mind.

Instead of choosing words that *can* convey what you mean, take the time to choose words that *precisely* convey what you mean.

Be picky. Own a dictionary and thesaurus (in print, on your phone, or on your computer) and consult them often. Consider the differences between similar words, and practice reading and editing your sentences until you get the words just right.

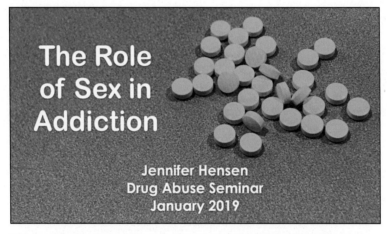

This is a title slide from a talk presented to scientists studying drug abuse and addiction. After reading the title, what do you think the talk was about? How sexual behavior influences drug use? How drug use influences sexual behavior? The talk was actually about how male and female rats differ in response to exposure to certain drugs of abuse. When choosing words for scientific presentations, try to choose words that convey the most information.

Try to avoid colloquialism and slang

Scientific writing has a reputation for being serious and dry. Even most scientists don't like professional scientific writing as an art form. As later chapters will discuss, serious writing need not be boring. But is it ever okay to be informal or colloquial with the words you choose?

In professional written presentations intended for other scientists, the answer is clearly no. Formal writing that becomes part of the scientific record should be free from colloquialism and slang.

Try to avoid:

- Contractions (e.g., can't, won't, don't).

- Colloquial phrases and idioms—informal language used by people in everyday speech:

    "On the other hand"

    "Take it with a grain of salt"

    "Cream of the crop"

    "Kill two birds with one stone"

- Slang—highly informal phrases:

    "Cutting edge"

    "Rock solid"

    "Cop out"

In poster presentations you have a little more freedom for informality (especially for non-professional, "in-house" poster sessions). Slide presentations can be the most informal of all. Depending on the venue, you can feel free to use contractions and more colloquial language. Just remember that the overarching goal is to communicate a message.

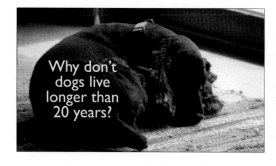
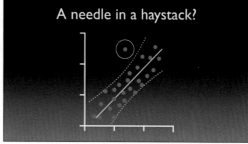

Avoid wordiness

In science presentations, there is usually an economy of words. Many journals insist on astonishingly low word limits, and slides and posters look best when you use as few words as possible. Therefore, brevity and clarity are paramount.

The best way to avoid wordiness is to carefully edit your sentences, omitting unnecessary words and shortening wordy phrases.

After writing a draft of a presentation, go through each sentence, one-by-one, and ask yourself if you can convey the same meaning with fewer words. Or even if you can omit words without replacing them and not losing meaning. For example, here are some common examples of wordy phrases in scientific writing:

Wordy	Concise
A total of …	*(Omit)*
All of …	All …
At the present time …	At present …
At this point in time …	At present …
Based on the fact that …	Because …
Both of …	Both …
During the course of …	During … or In …
Figure 1 shows that …	… (Figure 1)
For the purpose of …	For … or To …
Has been shown to be …	Is …
In light of the fact that …	Because …
In order to …	To …
In a small amount of …	Rarely … or Occasionally …
In previous years …	Previously …
In may be that …	Perhaps …
It should be mentioned …	*(Omit)*
It is interesting to note that	Of interest is …
More often than not …	Usually …
… quite unique	… unique
Really …	*(Omit)*
… small in size	… small
The reason is because …	The reason is …
… very …	*(Omit)*
… would seem to suggest …	… suggest …

Singular versus plural

To make most English words plural, you simply add the letter "−s." To make words that end in −ch, −x, or −s plural, you usually add an "−es." There are some exceptions for common English words, but there are many exceptions for words in science. Many scientific words maintain their original Latin or Greek form in plural, and their use may not seem intuitive or natural.

Single	Plural
Analysis	Analyses
Appendix	Appendices
Bacterium	Bacteria
Basis	Bases
Criterion	Criteria
Datum	Data
Focus	Foci
Genus	Genera
Homo sapiens	*Homo sapiens*
Hypothesis	Hypotheses
Index	Indices
Locus	Loci
Matrix	Matrices
Medium	Media
Nebula	Nebulae
Nucleus	Nuclei
Phenomenon	Phenomena
Serum	Sera
Species	Species
Symposium	Symposia
Thesis	Theses

Probably the most misused plural word in the list above is "data," which many people mistakenly use in reference to a single item. The word "data" should always be used as plural.

Incorrect	Correct
The data shows	The data show
The data suggests	The data suggest
The data supports …	The data support …
The data is not …	The data are not …

Choosing the active versus the passive voice

Be conscious about your use of the active versus the passive voice. In the active voice, the subject of the sentence *does* an action. In the passive voice, the subject *receives* an action.

Active: We stained the cells using immunohistochemistry.
Passive: The cells were stained using immunohistochemistry.

Both of these sentences are grammatically correct, but each sentence emphasizes different information. In the active voice, there is more emphasis placed on who is staining the cells. "We" is the subject of the sentence. In the passive voice, it is unknown who stained the cells. "Cells" is the subject of the sentence.

It is customary to use the passive voice in scientific writing even though the active voice is often more concise and provides more information. There are at least two reasons to use the passive voice: (1) The passive voice de-emphasizes *who* is doing the work and instead emphasizes the work being done. In science, the focus should be on the work, not the scientists conducting the experiments. (2) The passive voice prevents repetition. For example, consider the following passage from a scientific methods section:

We dissolved the Hcrt antagonist in artificial cerebrospinal fluid and stored aliquots at −20°C prior to use. We infused the antagonist bilaterally using a minipump at a rate of 0.1 μL/min for 3 min. We used the same injection coordinates used to deliver AAV5 above the LC region.

These sentences use the active voice, but they all start with "We …" and emphasize the scientists performing the experiments. In contrast, consider the same section with a mix of the active and passive voice:

We dissolved the Hcrt antagonist in artificial cerebrospinal fluid and stored aliquots at −20°C prior to use. Microinfusions were performed bilaterally using a minipump at a rate of 0.1 μL/min for 3 min. Injection coordinates were the same used to deliver AAV5 above the LC region.

There are no firm guidelines on whether the active or passive voice is best, except to be deliberate about which you choose throughout your presentation. Try to use the active voice as often as possible, but not at the expense of effective, non-repetitive writing.

Choosing verb tense

The verbs you use can be phrased in the past, present, or future tense. The future tense is obviously only used to describe potential or proposed actions/experiments that have not yet been performed. However, it is not immediately obvious when to use the past and present tenses in science communication. Scientists are not consistent. Open a single issue of a scientific journal and you may find inconsistencies among the use of the past and present tenses among the different articles.

In general, it is best to use the past tense to describe actions and experiments and the present tense to describe knowledge accepted as valid conclusions.

Always describe methods and actions of experiments (performed by you or others) in the past tense because these experiments took place in the past:

> We **collected** five specimens from each plant …
> Owen et al. (2005) **found** that …
> Each mouse **was implanted** with a 22G cannula …
> Two days later, all of the cells **were dead** and detached from the plate …

Describe the conclusions of experiments in the present tense because the conclusions don't change with time:

> Flies and mice **prefer** sweet compounds to bitter compounds …
> Owen et al. (2005) found that dogs **increase activity** after consuming sugars …
> Metal objects **conduct heat** more than wooden objects …
> A 50% ethanol solution **is** toxic to cells …

When writing a full research study, each section has optimal choices for past versus present verbs. An **Abstract** should contain both past and present verbs. Use the present tense to introduce relevant background information and the past tense to summarize what you did. An **Introduction** should mostly consist of information in the present tense. The present tense suggests your acceptance of the conclusions of past studies. Your **Methods** and **Results** should be in the past tense to describe the experients you performed in your recent study. A **Discussion** should be a mixture of past and present verbs to integrate what you found (in the past) with what is already known (accepted as current knowledge). Finally, a **Conclusion** should be in the present tense to place your findings in the context of the permanent scientific record.

Commonly misused or incorrect words

There are several words that scientists commonly misuse or that aren't optimal for certain meanings. There are even some commonly used words that don't even exist! Although a copy editor at a journal will no doubt find and correct these mistakes, peer reviewers or audience members may interpret sloppy word choice as carelessness and connoting unprofessionalism.

Adaption   *Adaption* is not a word. The correct word is *adaptation*.

As   Don't use *as* in place of the word *because*. *As* means *in the same way that* … or *at the moment that* … For example: "English as a second language," or "The egg cooked as the water boiled."

Comprise   The word *comprise* means *to contain*, as in "the solar system comprises the sun and planets. It does not mean *to constitute* or *to make up*.

Correlate to   Items/concepts might be related *to* each other, but they are always correlated *with* one another.

Could of   *Could of* is grammatically incorrect; the correct usage is *could have*.

Dilemma   *Dilemma* doesn't simply mean *a difficult problem* or a *quandary*. Instead, it means a decision between two equally good or bad choices.

Due to   The word *due* implies a debt or deadline. Therefore, don't use *due* when you mean to say *because of*.

Different than   Two items are different *from* each other, not different *than* each other.

Experience(d)   *Experience* implies sensation. Therefore, only use this word in reference to living, sensing creatures/objects, as opposed to statements like "the Earth experienced a cooling period," or "The forest experienced high winds."

Irregardless   Irregardless is not a word. Use *regardless.*

Literally   *Literally* means that *something is completely and totally true in a literal sense.* Because this word can be used for dramatic effect, sometimes people use it when they actually should use the word's exact opposite, *figuratively*, which means that something is not true in a literal sense.

Peruse   A common misconception is that *peruse* means *to browse or skim lightly.* It actually means the opposite: *to read with great care and attention to detail.*

Significant   In science presentations, only use *significant* in reference to statistical significance. When not describing statistics, consider using the words *substantial, notable,* or *remarkable.*

Since   Don't use *since* in place of the word *because.* Since connotes time, as in "I haven't seen you since this morning."

Thing   The word *thing* is okay to use when referring to an object, but many people use it to represent an abstract concept: "The thing I don't like about the paper ..."; "The thing I like about your proposal ..."; "Here's the thing ..." Try your best to be more specific. Use thing if you feel you have to, but more specific words force you to communicate better with a reader.

This   Don't use *this* in isolation. The problem with *this* is that it isn't descriptive enough. This just won't do. Instead, be specific: "This concept ...," "This question ...," "This phenomenon ...," etc.

Where   *Where* should always be used in reference to a location. Don't use *where* instead of *in which*, or *for which*. For example: "This is a protocol *in which* we need to pay careful attention to detail.

While   *While* should always be used in reference to time. Don't use *while* instead of *and, but, although,* or *whereas.* For example: "The inner planets are mostly rocky, whereas the outer planets are mostly gaseous."

Understanding the distinctions between similar words

The following words are often mistakenly interchanged. Make sure you know which is the correct word to use in a given context.

Affect versus Effect. Affect is always a verb, meaning *to influence or cause an effect.* **Effect** is most often used as a noun, meaning *a result.* It is also sometimes a verb, meaning *to bring about.*

> *How does the temperature **affect** the reaction?*
> *What is the **effect** of temperature on the reaction?*
> *We hope the results of this study will **effect** policy change.*

Appears versus Seems. Appears means *becoming visible* or *coming into view.* **Seems** means *giving the impression of being.*

> *Our paper **appears** on PubMed sometime this week.*
> *The data **seem** too good to be true.*

Compare to versus Compare with. Compare to means *to represent something as similar to something else.* **Compare with** means *to determine the similarities and differences.*

> *His level of strength **compares to** that of a much younger man.*
> *I think you should **compare** your results **with** the results of other studies.*

Denote versus Connote. Denote means *to designate* or *to indicate a primary meaning* to something. **Connote** means *to imply* or *to hint about characteristics* suggested by something.

> *Her status as a Nobel Laureate **denotes** that she was awarded a Nobel Prize.*
> *Her Nobel Prize **connotes** that she is an outstanding scientist.*

It's versus Its. It's is a contraction for *it is.* **Its** is the possessive form of *it.* Usually possessive words end with an apostrophe −s ('s), as in: "North America's contribution to greenhouse gas emissions." **Its** is an exception and never shows possession.

> *It's an undocumented species.*
> *The dog hurt **its** leg on the rocky trail.*

Imply versus Infer. Imply means *to insinuate* or *to suggest.* **Infer** means *to deduce* or *to conclude.* Presenters **imply**, audience members **infer**.

> *The politician **implied** that global warming is not real.*
> *I **infer** from your speech that you believe global warming is not real.*

Percentage versus Percent. Percentage is a noun meaning *an amount that is a proportion of a larger sum.* **Percent** is an adverb that always represents *a specified amount for every hundred.* **Percent** should always be used with a number.

> *What is the **percentage** of people who follow your blog overseas?*
> *Fifteen **percent** of Americans approve of Congress.*

Predominant versus Predominate. Predominant is an adjective meaning *principal, chief, controlling.* **Predominate** is a verb meaning *to be predominant* and/or *to be in the majority.*

> *My **predominant** objective in presenting this talk is to attract graduate students to my lab.*
> *Butterflies **predominate** over other species in this habitat.*

Principal versus Principle. Principal is either a noun meaning *a person in charge,* or an adjective meaning *most important.* **Principle** is a noun meaning *a rule, doctrine, or truth.*

> *She is the **principal** of the elementary school.*
> *The **principal** finding of this study is that the universe is expanding.*
> *The guiding **principle** of cell culture is to keep everything as sterile as possible.*

That versus Which. That and **which** both add additional information about the subject or object of a sentence. **That** usually does not follow a comma, and restricts or defines the meaning of something. **Which** almost always follows a comma, and adds additional information about the meaning of something.

> *The mice **that** had been raised in an enriched environment lived longer than mice **that** were isolated in cages without running wheels.*
> *The mice, **which** have a shorter lifespan than rats, were raised in either an enriched environment or in isolated cages.*

The burden of proof

When describing the conclusion of an experiment or study, your choice of words is very important to communicate the strength of your results. As scientists, we naturally want to promote our work by emphasizing the importance of scientific results. However, we also don't want to exaggerate our conclusions with language that is too strong.

Choose your words carefully about what your data show. Consider the possibility that future studies may present contradictory findings that challenge your conclusions.

The results...

...prove...	Strong conclusion
...unambiguously show...	
...show...	
...demonstrate...	
...indicate...	
...substantiate...	
...strongly suggest...	
...argue for...	
...suggest...	
...support...	
...are consistent with...	
...are compatible with...	Cautious conclusion
...are not inconsistent with...	

The meaning of Latin abbreviations

Latin was the universal academic language of Western civilization for several centuries. Although Latin is no longer a commonly spoken language, many Latin scientific terms remain in use, especially in abbreviated form.

C.V.   **Curriculum vitae:** *Course of life.* A document that lists all of the relevant education, training, jobs, and successes in one's career. Usually more extensive than a resume.

       I would be happy to consider you for a position if you send me your current C.V.

e.g.   **Exempli gratia:** *For example.* For example; for instance. Always use this term in a scientific presentation instead of "ex."

       You must obtain IACUC approval before doing experiments on vertebrate animals (e.g., mice or rats).

et al.   **Et alia:** *And others.* The other people who contributed; colleagues. In science, this term almost always applies to coauthors of a research study.

       Our results are consistent with the findings of Prolo et al. (2016).

etc.   **Et cetera:** *And other things.* Other people or items in the same category. Make sure to use at least two or more items preceding this term.

       There are many neuropeptides expressed in the brain, including hypocretin, kisspeptin, agouti-related protein, etc.

i.e.   **Id est:** *That is.* In other words …

       Many lizard species demonstrate metachrosal circadian rhythms, i.e., the ability to change body color throughout the day.

Guidelines for writing about numbers

Because of the speed with which we read text about numbers, sometimes it is best to write out numbers as words (e.g., sixteen, twenty-nine, forty-three), and other times it is best to write out numbers as numerals (16, 29, 43). Use the following guidelines to determine whether words or numerals are most appropriate for your sentences.

Write out single-digit whole numbers as words and use numerals for numbers greater than nine.

> *We used eight mice in this study.*
> *We used 26 mice in this study.*

Be consistent when writings words versus numerals for a category of information. If you choose to use numerals, use numerals for all numbers in that category. Likewise, if you choose to use words, use words for all numbers in that category.

> *This study consisted of 6 girls and 14 boys.*
> *We hoped to discover at least twenty new species, but only discovered three.*

Never start a sentence with a numeral. Try not to start a sentence with a number greater than ninety-nine.

> *Twenty-six mice were used in this study.*
> *Since the study began, we recruited over 1300 subjects.*

Use numerals to report statistics, provide quantitative data using units of measurement, and when describing dates, times, pages, figures, and tables.

> *Only 5% of neurons transduced with GFP showed co-expression with Fos (Figure 1).*
> *All stimulation episodes lasted 5 h (between 13:00 and 18:00).*

Write decimals as numerals and always place a zero in front of a number less than one.

> *The vehicle reached maximum velocity in 11.24 s.*
> *The water level rose 0.13 m last year.*

Always spell out simple fractions.

> *One-half of the mice were fed chow and one-half were fed sucrose pellets.*
> *Two-thirds of the students come from disadvantaged backgrounds.*

Express mixed fractions as numerals unless they begin a sentence.

> *The imaging procedure lasted 7 h.*
> *Seven and one-half hours later, the imaging was complete.*

Never place two numbers next to each other without a comma unless you write one as a numeral and one as a word (for different categories of information).

> *This study imaged thirteen 17-year-old males.*
> *The ages of the four subjects were 17, 29, 39, and 45.*

Hyphenate all compound numbers from twenty-one through ninety-nine.

> *Sixty-three adult males took part in the study.*

Spell out centuries and decades either as words or numerals. If you use words, write the century or decade in lowercase. If you use numerals, use an apostrophe for abbreviated decades but never between the number and the −s.

> *Scientists began using fMRI in humans in the nineties.*
> *Scientists began using fMRI in humans in the '90s.*
> *Scientists began using fMRI in humans in the 1990s.*

Summary: Design principles for word choice

- It is often possible to express the same idea using many combinations of words. Instead of choosing words that *can* convey what you mean, choose words that *precisely* convey what you mean.

- Avoid colloquialism and slang for written presentations and as much as possible in slide presentations.

- Avoid wordiness as much as possible. After writing a draft, carefully edit your sentences to omit unnecessary words and shorten wordy phrases.

- Be careful about how many science words are phrased in the singular versus plural, especially the word "data" (which is always plural).

- Try to achieve a harmony between the active and passive voice in scientific writing. Passive voice allows you to emphasize the science over the people who conducted the science.

- Use the past tense of verbs to describe actions and experiments performed in the past, while using the present tense to describe knowledge accepted as valid conclusions.

- When forming conclusions, choose your words carefully about what your data show. Consider the possibility that future studies may present contradictory findings and phrase your conclusions with caution.

- Follow guidelines when choosing to write numbers as numerals or as words to enhance the speed with which readers will perceive your writing.

6

Tables

Tables display data (numbers or words) organized in rows and columns. Unlike figures, tables usually show data in their unprocessed, rudimentary form. The key to designing a great table is to arrange information clearly and logically so that data are easily accessible and maximally comprehensible to an audience.

Designing Science Presentations. https://doi.org/10.1016/B978-0-12-815377-2.00006-8

When to use a table instead of text or a figure

Tables are beneficial because they allow you to present a large quantity of information that would be too tedious and cumbersome to present as text. For example, consider the following passage:

The minimum average monthly temperatures for Seattle, WA are: January, 2.4 °C; February, 2.8 °C; March, 2.6 °C; April, 4.9 °C; May, 7.6 °C; June, 10.9 °C; July, 12.6 °C; August, 12.8 °C; September, 10.5 °C; October, 7.8 °C; November, 4.8 °C; December, 2.6 °C. The maximum average monthly temperatures are: January, 6.1°C; February, 9.8 °C; March, 11.8 °C; April, 14.1°C; May, 17.7 °C; June, 20.8 °C; July, 22.7 °C; August, 22.8 °C; September, 19.7 °C; October, 16.1°C; November, 10.9 °C; December, 7.7 °C. The average monthly rainfall is: January, 142.2 mm; February, 88.9 mm; March, 94.0 mm; April, 68.8 mm; May, 48.3 mm; June, 40.6 mm; July, 17.8 mm; August, 22.9 mm; September, 38.1 mm; October, 88.9 mm; November, 167.6 mm; December, 137.2 mm.

Not only is this text cumbersome to read, it is very hard for a reader to access a particular value of interest, for example, the maximum average monthly temperature for Seattle in September. A table could provide the same information in a much more visibly accessible format.

Table 1. Average monthly minimum temperature, maximum temperature, and rainfall in Seattle, WA.

Month	Min Temp (°C)	Max Temp (°C)	Rainfall (mm)
January	2.4	6.1	142.2
February	2.8	9.8	88.9
March	2.6	11.8	94.0
April	4.9	14.1	68.8
May	7.6	17.7	48.3
June	10.9	20.8	40.6
July	12.6	22.7	17.8
August	12.8	22.8	22.9
September	10.5	19.7	38.1
October	7.8	16.1	88.9
November	4.8	10.9	167.6
December	2.6	7.7	137.2

Use a table instead of text when it is easier to access single values of information from much larger datasets.

In contract, a graph is much better than a table for visually conveying the differences, patterns, trends, or interactions between values.

Table 2. Food consumed (g) in five individuals following injection of compound JSB3341.

Mouse	Day 1	Day 2	Day 3	Day 4
1	8.2	10.9	10.2	8.0
2	7.4	9.6	11.9	10.0
3	11.3	10.6	11.5	11.5
4	10.5	12.4	16.5	19.2
5	6.9	7.8	7.2	7.5

The table on the left contains the same information as the graph below, however, the relationship between the data is more apparent and accessible in the graph.

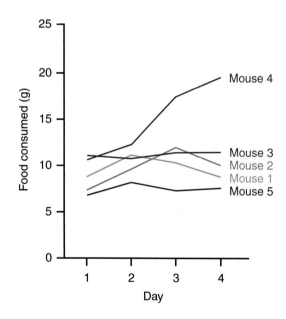

Anatomy of a table

Each scientific journal has its own guidelines for creating tables; however, all good tables share certain design elements.

A table should be completely comprehensible on its own. Information in a well-designed table should be easy to understand and access, even if the table is removed from the rest of a presentation.

The **title** of your table must adequately and completely describe the contents of the table. Usually the title is a sentence fragment (lacking a verb) written in sentence case (only the first letter is capitalized). Try to communicate as much information as possible.

Before   Injection coordinates
After   Injection coordinates of all brain regions targeted with AAV

Before   Planetary probes
After   Probes that have landed on other planets

Before   Lizards studied
After   Sex, weight, and snout-vent length of *Sceloporus malachiticus* individuals

Column titles must be short and specific. To make these titles shorter, it is usually okay to employ abbreviations that normally you wouldn't use (e.g., "temp" for temperature or "conc" for concentration).

Demarcation lines divide different parts of a table to help categorize information. These lines should be placed above and below column headings and at the very bottom of the table.

Footnotes describe or clarify information from the table in more detail. These are always placed immediately beneath the table.

Title

Table 3. Percentage of neurons co-expressing Fos following stimulation of Hcrt neurons after 0 or 4 h sleep deprivation.

Column titles

Cell group	0 h sleep deprivation		4 h sleep deprivation	
	No stim	Stim	No stim	Stim
Basal forebrain	4.14 +/- 5.27 n=674	44.21 +/- 7.22** n=721	3.24 +/- 5.46 n=677	4.99 +/- 1.98 n=702
DRN	8.94 +/- 3.48 n=315	9.33 +/- 3.00 n=345	6.29 +/- 2.76 n=308	9.04 +/- 3.84 n=361
Hcrt neurons	13.49 +/- 3.89 n=761	42.98 +/- 8.33** n=802	13.99 +/- 4.18 n=739	39.66 +/- 6.13** n=779
LC	12.24 +/- 4.16 n=881	39.24 +/- 8.74** n=932	17.94 +/- 4.01 n=975	21.14 +/- 4.75 n=953
MCH	3.45 +/- 1.55 n=821	2.21 +/- 1.23 n=783	2.98 +/- 1.01 n=756	3.11 +/- 0.87 n=801
TMN	11.87 +/- 4.98 n=289	23.44 +/- 6.24* n=320	11.06 +/- 2.69 n=351	13.21 +/- 4.52 n=340
VLPO	2.87 +/- 1.23 n=57	5.42 +/- 1.65 n=71	3.54 +/- 1.82 n=63	4.44 +/- 0.98 n=69
VTA	5.68 +/- 2.03 n=893	25.12 +/- 4.87** n=927	4.25 +/- 1.65 n=910	7.82 +/- 2.31 n=917

Data

Footnotes

Values represent the mean percentage of neurons (n) that also co-express Fos, +/- the standard error of the mean. Double asterisk, p<0.001; asterisk, p<0.05; two-tailed Student's t-test between Hcrt::mCherry and Hcrt::ChR2-mCherry transduced animals. Abbreviations: DRN, dorsal raphe nuclei; Hcrt, hypocretin; LC, locus coeruleus; MCH, melanin concentrating hormone neurons; TMN, tuberomammilary nucleus; VLPO, ventrolateral preoptic nucleus; VTA, ventral tegmental area.

Demarcation lines

Logically formatting a table

Categories of comparative data should be presented vertically in columns, not horizontally in rows.

Table 4. Area, length, and maximum depth of the three largest African lakes.

Lake	Malawi	Tanganyika	Victoria
Area (km^2)	30,044	32,893	69,485
Length (km)	579	676	322
Depth (m)	706	1470	84

Table 4. Area, length, and maximum depth of the three largest African lakes.

Lake	Area (km^2)	Length (km)	Depth (m)
Malawi	30,044	579	706
Tanganyika	32,893	676	1470
Victoria	69,485	322	84

Both tables present the same data, but the table on the right is organized more logically and is easier to read. The eye tends to read down columns more naturally than read across rows, so comparative statistics should be arranged vertically.

Use a hierarchical organization to emphasize the categories you think are most important.

Table 5. Number of men and women selected by NASA to be astronauts by year of selection.

	Men			Women		
	1980	1990	2000	1980	1990	2000
Mission specialist	9	12	7	2	4	3
Pilot	8	6	7	0	1	0
Total	17	18	14	2	5	3

Table 5. Number of men and women selected by NASA to be astronauts by year of selection.

	1980		1990		2000	
	Men	Women	Men	Women	Men	Women
Mission specialist	9	2	12	4	7	3
Pilot	8	0	6	1	7	0
Total	17	2	18	5	14	3

The table on the left emphasizes the comparison between men and women. The table on the right emphasizes the comparison between years of selection.

Horizontal entries of data should not be listed randomly. Order information in alphabetical or numerical order depending on which data you want to emphasize.

Table 6. Diameter and mass of planets in relation to the Earth.

Planet	Diameter	Mass
Mercury	0.38	0.06
Venus	0.95	0.82
Earth	1.00	1.00
Mars	0.53	0.11
Jupiter	11.21	317.80
Saturn	9.45	95.20
Uranus	4.01	14.60
Neptune	3.88	17.20

Table 6. Diameter and mass of planets in relation to the Earth.

Planet	Diameter	Mass
Earth	1.00	1.00
Jupiter	11.21	317.80
Mars	0.53	0.11
Mercury	0.38	0.06
Neptune	3.88	17.20
Saturn	9.45	95.20
Uranus	4.01	14.60
Venus	0.95	0.82

Table 6. Diameter and mass of planets in relation to the Earth.

Planet	Diameter	Mass
Jupiter	11.21	317.80
Saturn	9.45	95.20
Uranus	4.01	14.60
Neptune	3.88	17.20
Earth	1.00	1.00
Venus	0.95	0.82
Mars	0.53	0.11
Mercury	0.38	0.06

The table on the left lists the planets in order from the sun. The center table lists the planets in alphabetical order. The table on the right lists the planets in descending order of diameter. Any order is acceptable as long as it follows an understandable hierarchy and emphasizes the main point that you want to convey.

Text and number alignment

Be deliberate about aligning text and numbers within tables. Certain design choices optimize clarity and the ability to visually access information.

Table 7. Average mass and length of ten of the heaviest mammals.

Animal	Environment	Avg. mass (kg)	Avg. length (m)
Asian elephant	Terrestrial	4,150	6.8
Blue whale	Aquatic	110,000	25.5
Fin whale	Aquatic	57,000	20.6
Giraffe	Terrestrial	1,015	5.1
Gray whale	Aquatic	19,500	13.5
Hippopotamus	Terrestrial	1,800	4.0
Humpback whale	Aquatic	29,000	13.5
Sperm whale	Aquatic	31,250	13.3
Walrus	Terrestrial	944	2.8
White rhinocerus	Terrestrial	2,100	4.4

Do: Align the major items on the lefthand side of a table flush left | Align text entries in the center or flush left | Align whole numbers flush right | Align numbers with decimals or +/– symbols centered on the decimal point or +/–

Don't: Align the major items on the lefthand side flush right or center | Align text entries flush right | Align whole numbers center or flush left | Align numbers with decimals or +/– symbols in the center or flush left or right

Table 7. Average mass and length of ten of the heaviest mammals.

Animal	Environment	Avg. mass (kg)	Avg. length (m)
Asian elephant	Terrestrial	4,150	6.8
Blue whale	Aquatic	110,000	25.5
Fin whale	Aquatic	57,000	20.6
Giraffe	Terrestrial	1,015	5.1
Gray whale	Aquatic	19,500	13.5
Hippopotamus	Terrestrial	1,800	4.0
Humpback whale	Aquatic	29,000	13.5
Sperm whale	Aquatic	31,250	13.3
Walrus	Terrestrial	944	2.8
White rhinocerus	Terrestrial	2,100	4.4

Choosing to add gridlines on tables

In written and poster presentations, it is usually best to avoid using gridlines to separate rows and columns of information. Unhelpful grids are unnecessary and can be distracting.

Name	Data	Data	Data	Data
Item A	2.3	1.9	8.7	9.0
Item B	4.0	7.2	9.1	5.5
Item C	0.4	0.8	5.2	0.6
Item D	8.0	9.4	1.0	4.2
Item E	6.3	3.5	8.0	6.0

Name	Data	Data	Data	Data
Item A	2.3	1.9	8.7	9.0
Item B	4.0	7.2	9.1	5.5
Item C	0.4	0.8	5.2	0.6
Item D	8.0	9.4	1.0	4.2
Item E	6.3	3.5	8.0	6.0

Occasionally, especially in a large table, subtle gridlines can help guide the reader in a sea of numbers. If it is helpful, add light horizontal gridlines every three to five rows. Alternatively, add subtle gray shading every other row. There are no firm rules on when to use these gridlines, so only use them when you feel they would be beneficial.

Name	Data	Data	Data
Item A	2.3	1.9	8.7
Item B	4.0	7.2	9.1
Item C	0.4	0.8	5.2
Item D	8.0	9.4	1.0
Item E	6.3	3.5	8.0
Item F	0.5	1.7	3.8
Item G	7.0	1.4	9.2
Item H	1.6	0.3	8.1
Item I	4.7	9.2	3.5
Item J	9.1	4.8	3.2
Item K	7.1	4.2	3.3
Item L	8.0	2.8	4.7

Name	Data	Data	Data
Item A	2.3	1.9	8.7
Item B	4.0	7.2	9.1
Item C	0.4	0.8	5.2
Item D	8.0	9.4	1.0
Item E	6.3	3.5	8.0
Item F	0.5	1.7	3.8
Item G	7.0	1.4	9.2
Item H	1.6	0.3	8.1
Item I	4.7	9.2	3.5
Item J	9.1	4.8	3.2
Item K	7.1	4.2	3.3
Item L	8.0	2.8	4.7

Name	Data	Data	Data
Item A	2.3	1.9	8.7
Item B	4.0	7.2	9.1
Item C	0.4	0.8	5.2
Item D	8.0	9.4	1.0
Item E	6.3	3.5	8.0
Item F	0.5	1.7	3.8
Item G	7.0	1.4	9.2
Item H	1.6	0.3	8.1
Item I	4.7	9.2	3.5
Item J	9.1	4.8	3.2
Item K	7.1	4.2	3.3
Item L	8.0	2.8	4.7

In contrast to written and poster presentations, gridlines are ideal for slide presentations. Audience members have a harder time distinguishing between rows and columns on a projected slide. Adding subtle gridlines can help the eye track data among horizontal and vertical categories.

Before

Name	Data	Data	Data	Data
Item A	2.3	1.9	8.7	9
Item B	4	7.2	9.1	5.5
Item C	0.4	0.8	5.2	0.6

After

Name	Data	Data	Data	Data
Item A	2.3	1.9	8.7	9
Item B	4	7.2	9.1	5.5
Item C	0.4	0.8	5.2	0.6

Reduce table size for slide presentations

Tables in written presentations can serve as a reference for extensive quantities of information that a reader can peruse whenever necessary. In contrast, tables in slide and poster presentations need to be brief because the audience cannot keep track of a large amount of information during a real-time delivery.

Table 8. Population, area, and density of the top twelve most populous U.S. cities[a].

Rank	City	State	Population	Area (sq. mi)	Density (per sq. mi)
1	New York	New York	8,175,133	302.6	27,016.3
2	Los Angeles	California	3,792,621	468.7	8,091.8
3	Chicago	Illinois	2,695,598	227.6	11,843.6
4	Houston	Texas	2,099,451	599.6	3,501.4
5	Philadelphia	Pennsylvania	1,526,006	134.1	11,379.6
6	Phoenix	Arizona	1,445,632	516.7	2,797.8
7	San Antonio	Texas	1,327,407	460.9	2,880.0
8	San Diego	California	1,307,402	325.2	4,020.3
9	Dallas	Texas	1,197,816	340.5	3,517.8
10	San Jose	California	945,942	176.5	5,359.4
11	Jacksonville	Florida	821,784	747.0	1,100.1
12	Indianapolis	Indiana	820,235	361.4	2,270.2

[a]Data from the 2010 United States Census.

The table on top is perfect for a written presentation, however, it could overwhelm an audience when used in a slide (as in the bottom left). The table in the slide at bottom right is highly accessible to an audience, but might be too simple for a written presentation.

Summary: Design principles for tables

- Tables are useful for showing a large quantity of information that would be too cumbersome to present as text. Graphs are more useful than tables for showing relationships between data.

- Tables are composed of informative titles, column titles, demarcation lines, footnotes, and of course your data.

- Tables can be designed to optimize clarity and legibility. Be deliberate about how you format your table, including how you align the text and numbers within your tables.

- Reduce the size of tables for slide presentations versus written presentations, because your audience won't be able to keep track of such detailed information.

7

Graphs

Graphs visually depict quantitative trends and relationships between different sets of data. Figures about quantitative data are the core of scientific presentations. Many audience members equate your quantitative figures with your results themselves, entirely judging the science you present by the information contained in your graphs. In research articles and posters, quantitative figures are often the first, and sometimes the only parts actively viewed by readers. Therefore, designing quality graphs is extremely important. As with the design of any aspect of a presentation, well-designed graphs communicate meaningful information in the simplest, clearest way possible.

Designing Science Presentations. https://doi.org/10.1016/B978-0-12-815377-2.00007-X

When to use a graph

Graphs are used to visually communicate patterns or trends within a specific dataset and to communicate differences or interactions among multiple categories of data. A graph is the most fundamental unit of a scientific presentation, representing a single aspect of a study with its own rationale, methods, and conclusions.

Well-designed graphs are inherently more interesting than text or tables because they not only present data, they also communicate meaningful relationships between data.

Use a graph to visually communicate patterns, trends, or relationships among data.

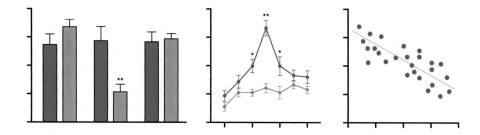

Consider not using a graph if there is no interesting trend in the data, or if there is no relationship between different categories of data. Also consider not using a graph if the data are too sparse to justify using a graph over words alone. Use the text or your oral narration to report sparse data, or tables to present complex datasets in which you do not need to highlight differences or trends.

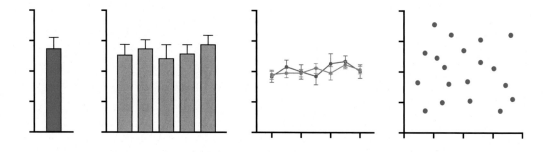

Anatomy of a graph

Audiences naturally focus on figures more than written text or oral narration. Therefore, well-designed graphs should ideally be comprehensible on their own, without the need for many supporting details found elsewhere.

Each category of graph has its own design considerations, however, the design goal for any graph is the same: to clearly convey the most information in the simplest, most accessible way possible.

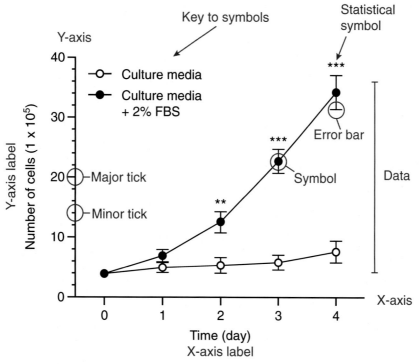

Figure legend

Figure 1. Addition of 2% fetal bovine serum (FBS) to culture medium increases the growth of DK cells. Data represent the mean +/- standard deviation; n=6 trials; **p<0.05, ***p<0.0001, repeated measures ANOVA followed with Bonferroni post hoc tests.

Categories of graphs

The five most common categories of graphs in science presentations are line graphs, bar graphs, histograms, scatterplots, and pie charts.

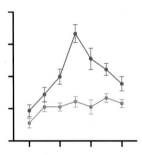

Line graph
Visualizes a trend of continuous data, often over time

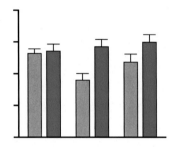

Bar graph
Compares discrete quantities of non-continuous data

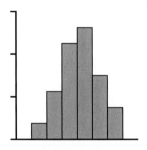

Histogram
Reports the distribution of data and the frequency with which they occur

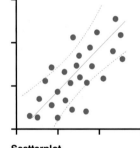

Scatterplot
Displays the relationship between two continuous variables

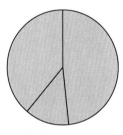

Pie chart
Shows the proportional values that make up a whole

Many other forms of charts exist that may better represent more specialized datasets.

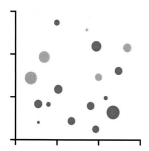

Bubble scatterplot
Displays the relationship between two continuous variables and a third variable represented by color and/or size

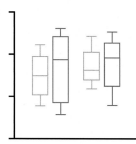

Box and whisker graph
Compares the maximum, upper quartile, median, lower quartile, and minimum values of one or more datasets

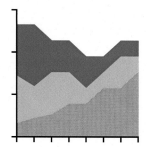

Area chart
Represents the cumulative totals of multiple, continuous data series, often over time

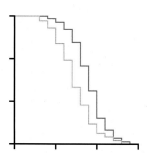

Decay/growth graph
Reports the cumulative decay or growth of one or more populations over time

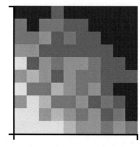

Heat map
Displays the relationship between two variables and the intensity of a third variable represented by a gradient of color

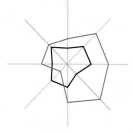

Radar chart
Compares values between two or more data series across multiple variables

General design considerations for graphs

Many scientists create graphs by entering data into spreadsheet programs and then letting the software make the graphs for them. Unfortunately, the default settings of many of these applications do not produce well-designed graphs, and even the software with the best default settings may not produce optimal graphs for your particular needs. Never trust a computer to do all of the design work for you. Instead, deliberately choose the colors, fonts, lines, and legends you use to visually communicate data in the most clear, understandable, and uncluttered way possible.

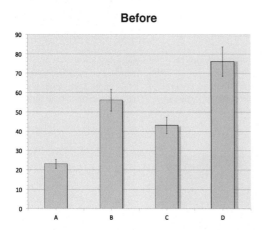

This graph was produced using the default settings on a standard spreadsheet graph-making program.

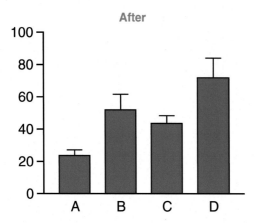

This graph was produced using the same data as above, however, every aspect of the graph was custom designed. All of the visual elements including the background color, the axes colors, the color of the bars, the absence of gridlines, the scale of the tick marks, the font, and the representation of error were deliberately chosen to optimize clarity.

Each kind of graph you make will require its own design considerations, however, there are some general principles that are usually consistent across different graph styles and different datasets:

Background color. Don't choose a special color for a graph background (the area created by the X- and Y-axes). Just use the same background as your presentation format. For written presentations, this will almost always be white.

Axes color. The color of the lines that make up your axes and tick marks should allow for the highest contrast with your background. If your background color is white or light in value, make your axes black. Likewise, if your background color is black or dark in value, make your axes white.

Color of datasets. The colors you choose to represent your data depend on many factors. Ideally, different datasets should contrast well with each other so that they are easy to visualize and compare with each other. Use a warmer color (e.g., red, yellow) to represent data that you especially want to emphasize. Whichever colors you choose, try to keep those colors consistent across your entire presentation so your audience has an easier time associating specific colors with specific categories of data.

Gridlines. In line graphs or bar graphs, only use gridlines if you need them. They are often unnecessary, but consider using them if you want your audience to perceive specific values of data that would be difficult to identify without grids.

Pleasing increments of scale. Some of the values you may assign as tick marks on your axes are inherently easier for audiences to grasp than others. Use increments that people naturally use when counting, such as multiples of 2, 5, 10, 20, 25, 100, etc. Avoid less-natural increments, such as multiples of 3, 4, 6, 12, 15, 75, etc.

Font. The fonts on graphs that are easiest to read are sans serif fonts with no overt personality (see Chapter 4). Helvetica or Arial are always good choices.

Representing error/variability. Show error/variability (such as the standard deviation or standard error of the mean) in a way that does not clutter your graph. Design error lines that are easy for your audience to see, but that don't overwhelm the actual data.

Representing significance. When choosing a symbol to represent significant differences between different categories of data, an asterisk is usually preferable over other symbols (e.g., %, #, &, @) that have other meanings. If you want to represent different significance values in the same graph, use repetitions of the same symbol (e.g., *, **, ***) rather than two or more different symbols so that the reader does not have to consult a figure legend to determine the relative strength of values.

Designing line graphs

Line graphs are used to display continuous data series and show trends over time. Often the most interesting conclusions in these graphs are about how the data change over time, or how different categories of data compare with each other, as opposed to the discrete values of the data themselves.

Before · **After**

To take full advantage of the size of your graph, the range in height of your data should ideally take up about three-fourths the height of the Y-axis. It is okay to not start the Y-axis at zero as long as your origin is clearly labeled.

To help your audience visualize discrete values of data, choose line weights that are about half as big as the data symbols themselves. Choose even lower line widths for the error bars.

Dashed lines are hard to read. To increase the contrast between two different categories of data, use different colors or shades.

Alternatively, vary the symbols used to represent data. It is usually easiest to distinguish between closed and open symbols (● versus ○) rather than different shapes (● versus ■).

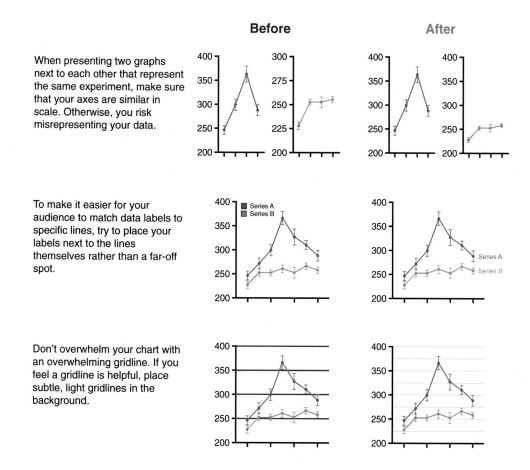

When presenting two graphs next to each other that represent the same experiment, make sure that your axes are similar in scale. Otherwise, you risk misrepresenting your data.

To make it easier for your audience to match data labels to specific lines, try to place your labels next to the lines themselves rather than a far-off spot.

Don't overwhelm your chart with an overwhelming gridline. If you feel a gridline is helpful, place subtle, light gridlines in the background.

To optimize clarity in a single graph, keep the maximum number of lines to about three or four. If you need more (or if your lines look crowded), separate your graphs into multiple panels.

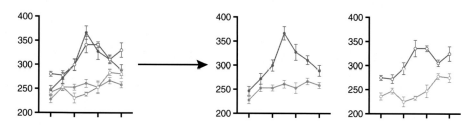

Designing bar graphs

Bar graphs are used to compare discrete quantities of non-continuous data.

Before   **After**

In most cases it is best to start the Y-axis of a bar chart at zero. Because the height of a bar represents a discrete value, charts that don't start at zero can be misleading. The exception is for data in which zero does not specify a value of "nothing," but exists on a relative continuum, for example, when measuring temperature.

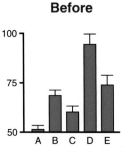 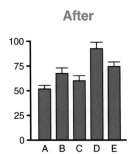

Don't let the thickness of the lines outlining the bars overwhelm the bars themselves. The most visible, prominent bars are contained within lines that are very fine but visible.

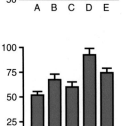 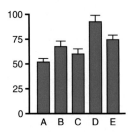

To increase visiblity of the individual bars, avoid bar widths that are too thin or thick. If the bars are too spread out, it can be more difficult to visually relate them to each other. The ideal spacing between bars is usually about one-third their width.

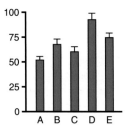 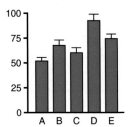

To help readers visualize different categories of data, don't place individual bars directly next to each other.

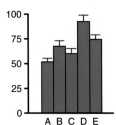 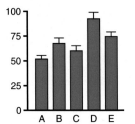

In bar charts with two or more categories of data, place a larger space between the different variables on the X-axis than between the different bars. Be sure to keep the order of the bars consistent across the X-axis.

Don't let statistical information overwhelm a graph. Show statistical differences between two bars using a thin line with subtle overhangs to aid the viewer's eye.

Place keys to data categories either to the right or on the top of a bar graph. If possible, the best way to save space is to place the key within the area of the bar graph itself.

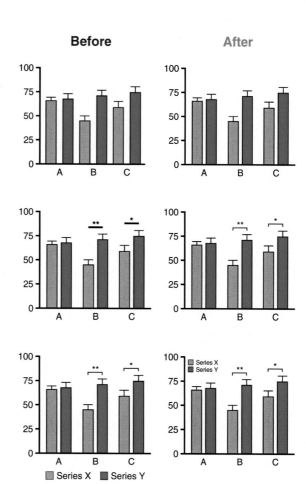

Before

After

Communicating maximum information in bar graphs

Bar graphs, by themselves, don't actually communicate much information except for discrete numbers, or the mean of a dataset with a representation of error. Consider communicating more information about datasets by superimposing visual information on top of the bars.

In a typical bar graph, the only infomation communicated by the bars themselves is the mean and error/variation of a group of data.

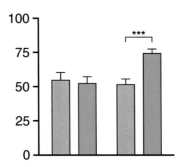

Depending on the amount of datapoints that contribute to each bar, you may be able to superimpose individual values on top of the bars to give readers a better sense of the entire dataset.

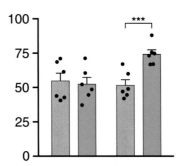

If adjacent bars are paired (the values represent the same subjects over different conditions or different times), consider connecting the datapoints across bars to show the individual changes.

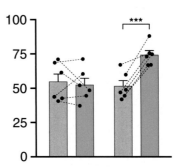

Superimposing several individual datapoints over bars and error bars may overwhelm a bar graph.

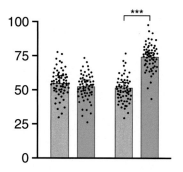

Therefore, it may be advantageous to remove the bar entirely and display only a "whisker" plot to show the mean and a measure of variation superimposed over several individual datapoints.

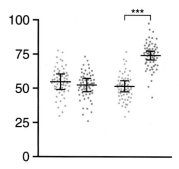

You might also summarize several datapoints using a box and whisker plot, which shows the maximum, upper quartile, median, lower quartile, and minimum values of one or more datasets

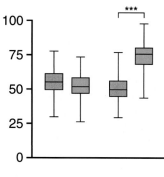

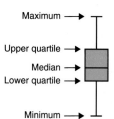

Designing histograms

A histogram shows the distribution of data and the relative frequency with which they occur.

Before **After**

Group data into separate "bins" to increase the clarity of the overal trend and reduce the effects of outliers.

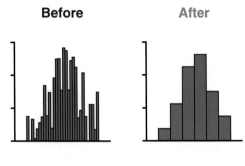

Depending on your data, it is usually best to have at least five bins. It is harder for readers to make conclusions about a dataset in a histogram with four or fewer bins.

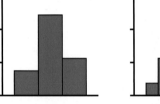 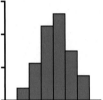

Don't unnecessarily assign different colors to different bins. If the histogram represents a single dataset, use the same color for all bins throughout.

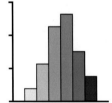 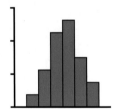

Before   **After**

Don't use spacing between bars on a histogram as you would on a bar chart. For frequency data, it is usually easier to perceive data as part of a unified dataset when the bars are placed directly adjacent to each other.

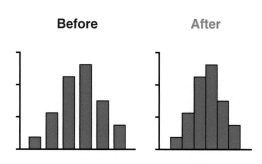

In contrast, use spacing between bars if there are two or more datasets plotted on the same histogram so that it is easier for readers to identify the bin value of each pair of bars...

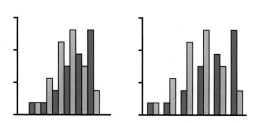

...however, notice above that plotting two or more datasets on the same histogram makes it much more difficult to perceive trends in the data. If it is necessary to plot two datasets together, consider filling in the body of one dataset while outlining the other. Alternatively, the clearest way to show two separate datasets is simply to plot them separately.

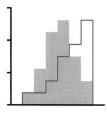
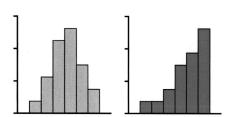

Designing scatterplots

Scatterplots are used to show the relationship between two continuous variables.

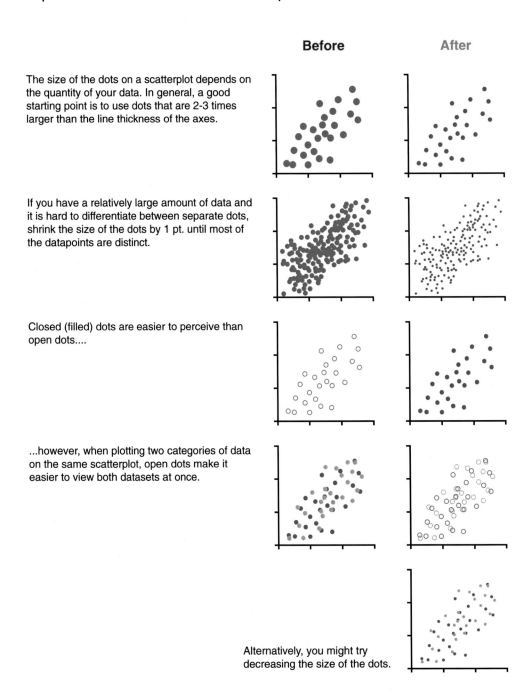

Before **After**

The size of the dots on a scatterplot depends on the quantity of your data. In general, a good starting point is to use dots that are 2-3 times larger than the line thickness of the axes.

If you have a relatively large amount of data and it is hard to differentiate between separate dots, shrink the size of the dots by 1 pt. until most of the datapoints are distinct.

Closed (filled) dots are easier to perceive than open dots....

...however, when plotting two categories of data on the same scatterplot, open dots make it easier to view both datasets at once.

Alternatively, you might try decreasing the size of the dots.

When you want to help your audience determine specific values of the individual datapoints, be cognizant about not overwhelming your scatterplot with distracting gridlines. Instead, place subtle gridlines in the background.

Use a line of best fit to represent a statistical statement about the relationship between the variables. Make sure the line stands out from the individual dots but does not overwhelm the scatterplot. Place statistical values somewhere on the chart where they do not clutter the data.

Consider using subtle lines to show other statistical parameters, such as 95% confidence intervals.

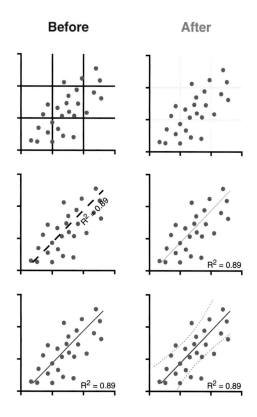

Scatterplots show the relationship between two continuous variables, but you can visualize a third variable by altering the color of the dots, or, in a bubble scatterplot, by altering the size of the dots.

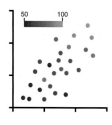

Depict a third, continuous variable via the color of the dots.

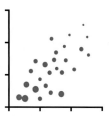

Depict a third, continuous variable via the area of the dots.

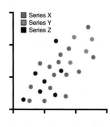

Depict different datasets via discrete colors of dots.

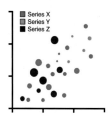

Depict different datasets via discrete colors of dots and a third, continuous variable via the area of the dots.

Designing pie charts

Use a pie chart to show relative proportions of a whole. Pie charts are not as good as bar graphs for showing absolute amounts or variability between data, however, they are sometimes better than bar charts for visualizing how constituent values add up to 100%.

Before   **After**

Try to start the largest slice of a pie chart at the 12:00 position. Usually it is easiest for audiences to perceive the relative proportions of the slices if the largest slice runs to the right of the 12:00 position, the second largest slice runs to the left of the 12:00 position, and the rest of the slices descend in value counter-clockwise.

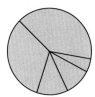 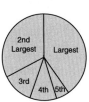

Assigning dark shades, bright hues, or multiple colors for different slices in a pie chart can distract your audience from the data within the chart. If it is necessary to apply different shades or colors (for example, when keeping different categories of data consistent from figure to figure), choose monochromatic colors, as described in Ch. 3, and try not to use distracting hues.

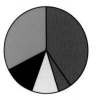 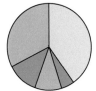

It is difficult for people to perceive differences between the sizes of slices if there are more than five or six slices. Otherwise, the visual distinction between different slices becomes meaningless.

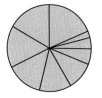 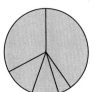

An exception occurs if you wish to highlight a single slice relative to all of the other slices in the pie.

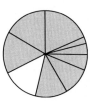

Designing Science Presentations

Try not to highlight more than one or two slices or to use highlighting colors that overwhelm the rest of the pie chart.

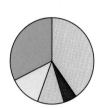

An alternative to highlighting a single slice with color is to use an "exploded pie" to emphasize a single slice. Don't use this method to emphasize more than one slice at a time.

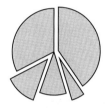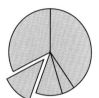

Instead of using a separate key (as you would for a line or bar graph), label the slices directly. If your label won't fit on the pie, place it immediately adjacent to the slice.

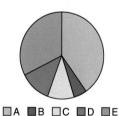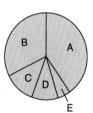

□A ■B □C ▨D ▧E

If you want to label each slice with the exact value or percentage of the whole, do so directly on the slice and not in a separate legend.

A: 42.0
B: 32.0
C: 12.0
D: 10.0
E: 4.0

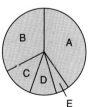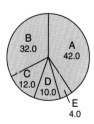

Help your audience visualize what is most important

Graphs are not only about axes and numbers, they are about relationships between different data. With some deliberate design decisions, you can help your audience visually understand what you find to be the most meaningful.

Design your charts so that readers will immediately visualize different categories of data and the relationships between them.

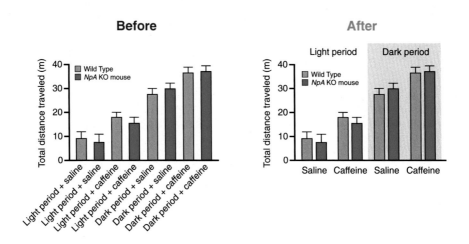

When appropriate, highlight data points that are particularly meaningful to you.

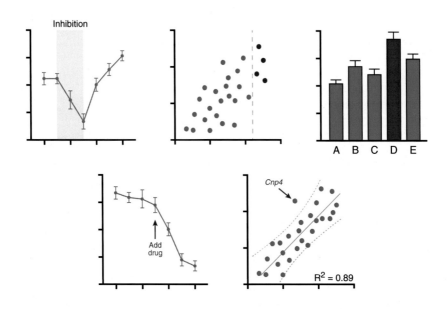

Reduce clutter, decoration, and distractions

Another way to help your audience visualize what is most important is to remove visual details that don't add information or meaning. Design graphs so that your content is the main feature and avoid the temptation to add decorative elements that distract from your main message.

The chart on the right is more clear because the serif font has been changed to sans serif and the shadow behind the bars has been removed.

In the chart on the left, the gradient isn't necessary. Additionally, the length of the tick marks is too long relative to the size of the chart.

Error bars on bar charts only need to be placed above the bar. If you want to emphasize that there is no significant difference between two sets of data, "n.s." can be useful. However, in many cases, it is only necessary to emphasize when there is a significant difference.

Many presenters think that 3D graphs look more professional and exciting than 2D. In reality, 3D charts contain awkward corners, shadows, and viewing angles that obscure the representation of data and cause difficulties in interpretation.

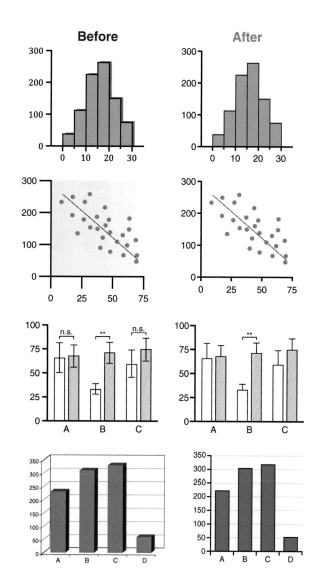

Use figure legends to convey supporting details

Figure legends provide detailed information that would be too visually cumbersome if placed within the graph itself.

Information to include in a figure legend includes:

- A specific title (written presentations only)

- Definitions as to what various symbols and shapes represent, including datapoints and scalebars

- Definitions of abbreviations

- *n* values, including the number of subjects, trials, sessions, etc.

- Definitions of statistical significance and reporting of statistical tests used

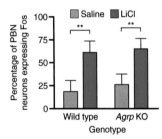

Figure 2. Intraperitoneal administration of LiCl causes an increase in the percentage of PBN neurons expressing Fos in both wild type and *Agrp* KO mice. n=8 animals per condition; **p<0.001, two-way ANOVA between genotype and treatment followed by Tukey posthoc test. AgRP, agouti-related protein; PBN, parabrachial nucleus.

Detailed figure legends are best used in written presentations. In slides or posters, minimal footnotes about a figure are best expressed in an abbreviated form beneath the figure in a way that does not detract from the figure itself.

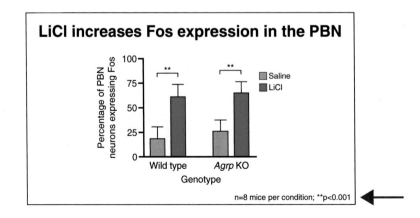

The best graph titles are often conclusions

Because well-designed graphs should stand on their own, the clearest, most direct titles are usually conclusions about the data. Although critical readers will evaluate a graph and draw their own conclusions, make it easy for them to understand what *you* conclude and want to say about your data.

The best graph titles not only describe experiments, they communicate the meaning of the results.

Before   Mass of rats over time

After   Rats on a high fat diet increase mass over time compared with rats fed normal chow

Before   Annual income versus socioeconomic background

After   Annual income positively correlates with socioeconomic background

Before   Effects of microstimulation of FEF on visual perception

After   Microstimulation of the FEF increases performance on a visual perception task

Before   Flies lacking *Smu2*

After   *Smu2*-null flies show no preference for sucrose versus quinine

Before   Average annual rainfall in Seattle during the 1990s

After   Average annual rainfall in Seattle remained stable during the 1990s

Before   Three-year prognosis after treatment

After   Increase in survival rate 3 years after treatment

Stating conclusions about a graph is not always possible or appropriate. For example, if presenting data about average monthly temperatures in North America, it probably isn't necessary to say, "Summer months are warmer than cooler months." However, this statement probably isn't the main, take-home point of the graph in the first place. Think of graph titles as an opportunity to say something important ... if a conclusion isn't suitable for your data, then let the graph speak for itself!

As stated in various other chapters, graph titles are placed in different locations in various presentation formats. In written documents, graph titles belong in the figure legends. In slide and poster presentations, graph titles are placed above the graphs themselves.

Summary: Design principles for graphs

- Well-designed graphs are inherently more interesting than text or tables because they not only present data, they also communicate meaningful relationships between data.

- Use a graph to visually communicate patterns, trends, or relationships among data. Consider using the text, a table, or oral narration to communicate sparse data, complicated data, or data in which there are no meaningful differences or trends.

- There are many common graphs used throughout the sciences, including line graphs, bar graphs, histograms, scatterplots, and pie charts; however, there are many other categories of graphs that may be optimal for specific datasets.

- Each category of graph has its own design considerations, however, the design goal for any graph is the same: to clearly convey the most information in the simplest, most accessible way possible.

- Don't trust the default settings of spreadsheet or graphing applications to do all of the design work for you. Instead, deliberately choose the colors, fonts, lines, and legends you use to visually communicate data in the most clear, understandable, and uncluttered way possible.

- Help your audience to visualize what is most important in your graphs by making design choices that maximize understanding and by highlighting data points that are particularly meaningful.

- Reduce clutter, decoration, and distractions in your graphs as much as possible. Avoid the temptation to add decorative elements that distract from your main message.

- Although graphs should be able to immediately convey a trend or relationship visually on their own, use figure legends to provide detailed information that would be too visually cumbersome if placed within the graph itself.

- The best graph titles are conclusions that communicate the meaning of the results.

8

Diagrams

Good diagrams are powerful visual tools that communicate information faster and often more thoroughly than text alone. They can quickly show how something works, how individual components make up a whole, how multiple items interact, and how events are ordered in time and space. Historically, scientific diagrams were predominantly created by professionals at scientific journals because scientists themselves didn't have the tools to create illustrations quickly. Now any scientist can create illustrations in a variety of software applications, and many journals even require authors to submit "summary diagrams" along with their manuscripts. They key to designing a good diagram is to always be conscious of its purpose, to help your audience understand a concept in the clearest, most straightforward way possible.

Designing Science Presentations. https://doi.org/10.1016/B978-0-12-815377-2.00008-1

When to use a diagram

Good diagrams present information in visual form, conveying concepts more quickly and clearly than words alone.

Use a diagram when it is more effective and/or expeditious to visually communicate a concept compared to communicating using words or verbal explanation.

There are many instances in science presentations in which it may be optimal to use a diagram:

- When conveying a "big picture" concept to an audience
- When showing a pictorial model of a research specimen or process of interest
- When visually conveying experimental strategies, methods, or techniques
- When sorting data or concepts into different categories
- When proposing a model

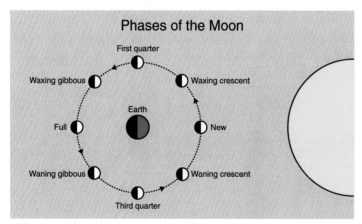

Imagine trying to convey the information in this diagram using text or oral explanation alone. Although possible, a diagram greatly helps the audience visualize information and discern how individual components of a process fit together into a whole.

Well-designed diagrams don't have to be artistic or flashy ... in fact, sometimes the most clear and elegant diagrams are composed of only the basic shapes, lines, arrows, and labels required to communicate a direct message. Don't worry if you feel unskilled or untalented in being able to create a diagram ... just think of the concepts you want to convey, and the process of making good design choices will likely lead you to a good outcome.

Clearly define the purpose of a diagram

The key to creating a good diagram is to start by clearly defining what you want your audience to understand. During the design process, add enough information to fully communicate what you want readers to understand while subtracting anything unnecessary.

Before starting to create a diagram, try finishing the prompt, "I want my audience to understand that .... " Doing so will help you focus on what visual elements you need to include and also what elements are *not* necessary to include.

Here is the first attempt at a diagram created in response to a prompt of "I want my audience to understand that chromosomal crossover occurs when two homologous chomosomes align and recombine."

This version presents not only the before and after conditions, but the intermediate step, which seems helpful to show.

This final version allows the reader to see the homologous recombination events with just enough labels for understanding. Many more labels might overwhelm the diagram and, depending on the audience, may not be necessary.

Homologous chromosomes

Chromosome crossover

Recombinant chromosomes

Showing relationships and sequence order in diagrams

When composing a diagram, decide how your visual elements relate to each other. What elements are the most important? How do they relate to other items? What order of information do you want readers to follow as they look at your diagram?

By using some simple design strategies, you can influence how readers perceive the hierarchies and relationships of the visual elements in your diagrams.

If certain elements in your diagram are more important than others, visually emphasize these elements using a different tint/shade, color, shape, size, or location.

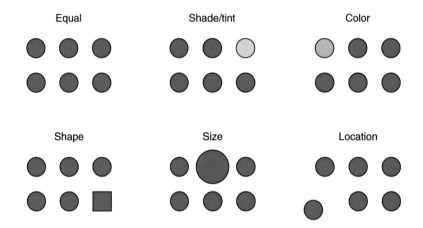

Consider the importance of the relationships between visual elements. Choose whether upstream or downstream elements are the most important and emphasize specific connections by the weights of arrows or lines.

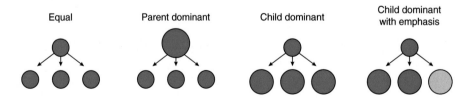

Also consider the order of information in your diagram. In Western cultures, we learn to read left to right, top to bottom. Therefore, audiences will find it easy and natural to read information in this order.

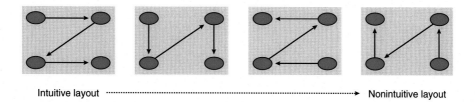

Intuitive layout ···▶ Nonintuitive layout

Many excellent diagrams work at an unconscious level … readers find them very clear and easy to read, unaware that they were deliberately designed to convey a sense of hierarchy, relationships, and logical order.

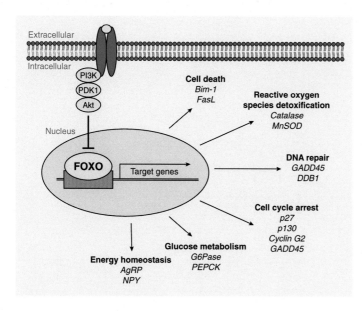

In this diagram, the visual element labeled "FOXO" is emphasized most, both in size and color. The audience has a clear sense of the flow of information (top to bottom, left to right) and that FOXO causes the activation of many distinct processes, all of which are emphasized equally. How would you design this figure differently if you wanted to emphasize the role of FOXO in cell cycle arrest?

Considerations for labeling diagrams

In many diagrams, visual elements often need to be labeled so that your audience knows the meaning of abstract drawings and symbols. Ideally, the labels should be secondary to the visual elements themselves and should not add too much clutter or distraction to a diagram.

Before   **After**

Don't force labels to fit inside visual elements. If an object is too small for a label, place the label just outside.

In contrast, place a label inside larger visual objects so it is easy to associate the label and the object.

If you need to use lines to connect your labels to the visual objects they identify, try not to use lines that are too thick. Also try not to cross the lines, or to let the lines cross through other objects.

To make your diagram more symmetrical and aesthetically pleasing, align multiple labels flush left or flush right towards the visual objects they identify.

When you obtain diagrams from other sources (e.g., a colleague, a research paper, the internet), there are often many more labels than you need for your own presentations. Adapt the image as your own (while acknowledging that you adapted the image and citing the source material), and only include labels as you would have done if you had created the diagram yourself.

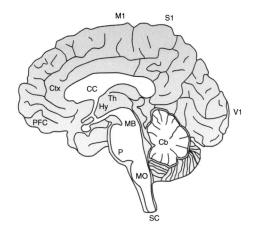

Before

The labels on this diagram initially served a useful purpose. However, for a talk about a specific brain structure, the multiple labels add distraction and clutter. With modern slide or photo editing software, it is relatively simple to erase or cover up these labels and to replace them with labels that are better suited to your needs.

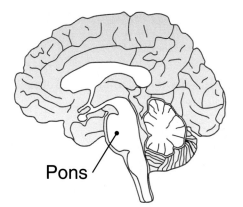

After

By only labeling the structure you care about, you remove distractions and the audience focuses on what is most important.

Designing Venn diagrams

Venn diagrams visualize the composition of two to five datasets and the degree to which they overlap. Each set is represented by a circle or ellipse, and the overlap shows what the sets share in common. Most Venn diagrams show two or three sets, but it is actually possible to show four or five.

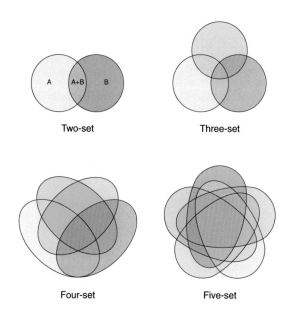

When representing quantitative data, ensure that numerical values are represented by the *area* of a circle rather than the radius or diameter.

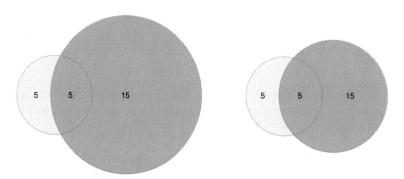

In these Venn diagrams, the yellow circle is meant to represent a total value of 10, the peach circle is meant to represent a total value of 20, and both circles are meant to overlap with a value of 5. Which is correct? Unfortunately, the diagram on the left represents the values of the data as the diameters of the circles, which is incorrect. As a result, the peach circle is much larger than it should be... over twice the size of the yellow circle. The diagram on the right correctly represents the data as the areas of the circles, and the peach circle is exactly twice as large as the yellow circle.

Designing flowcharts

A flowchart is a visual representation of a decision-making process. The first item in a flowchart often starts with a problem or question. Various steps along the chart require a decision, which eventually leads to a solution or end result. These diagrams are excellent for showing audiences your experimental methodology, such as what you will do following one of multiple experimental outcomes.

To help your audience visualize the various steps in a flowchart, use different shapes and/or colors to represent different types of nodes in the decision-making process.

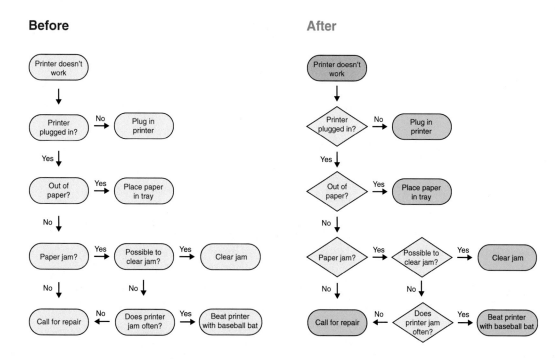

In the flowchart on the left, the nodes and text are clear, but it is harder to understand the important decision making points. In contrast, the flowchart on the right represents the problem as a pink oval, represents the decision making nodes as blue diamonds, and represents the potential outcomes as green ovals. Even without reading the labels, it is possible to determine the beginnings, middles, and ends of the flowchart.

Designing tree diagrams

Tree diagrams are used to show linear relationships between items. These relationships are often chronological or hierarchical.

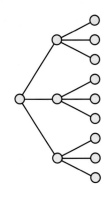

When describing cause-and-effect relationships or relationships that take place over time, it is usually most intuitive to perceive relationships from left to right.

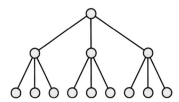

When representing hierarchy, it is usually most intuitive to perceive retionships from top to bottom.

When creating a tree diagram, consider whether you can represent the strength of the relationships between different items by the lengths of the lines connecting them. For example, this phylogenetic tree diagram represents the evolutionary relationship of different organisms. The longer the distance between two elements, the more they are evolutionarily divergent.

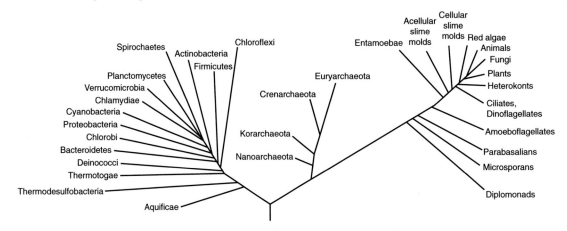

Designing timelines

Timelines show the temporal relationships between discrete events. They are especially great tools for visualizing the order of events in an experiment or conveying historical background information.

The most common mistake people make when designing timelines is to let words, arrows/lines, and/or symbols become too crowded and overwhelming. To help declutter a timeline, use the space above and below a timeline to separate information. Also consider employing different colors to group information into categories.

Before **After**

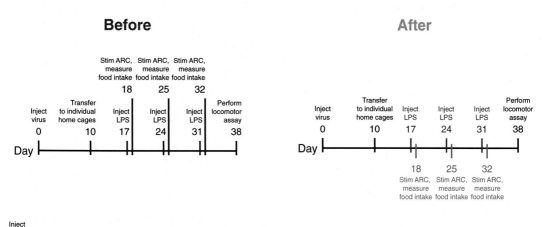

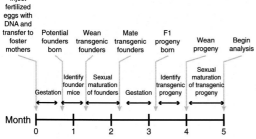
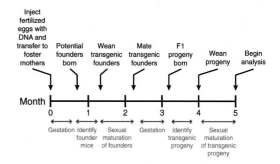

Designing pictorial diagrams

Pictorial diagrams visualize the component parts of real, physical objects/entities.

Don't feel intimidated about composing a pictorial diagram if you don't feel you have drawing skills. The most important feature of a good pictorial diagram is the clarity of the information, not the quality of the drawing.

In fact, perhaps the most common mistake in representing objects is to include too much detail in the drawing. These diagrams are not intended to be works of fine art, they are designed to communicate information.

Some general tips:

- Don't feel you have to reinvent the wheel! Many scientific concepts are commonly represented in images online, in textbooks, and in published papers. Try to find a few good images for inspiration, sketch out the best attributes of these images in your own way, and then determine what you need to add/subtract for your own needs.

- Only draw visual aspects that are necessary for the audience to identify structures or communicate information.

- Use the fewest number of colors possible. Note how the example diagrams on these pages each use two or three colors. Using more colors than necessary only complicates the diagram.

- Try not to overwhelm a picture with labels. Only identify structures that are necessary to show your audience.

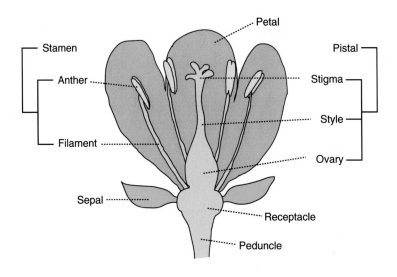

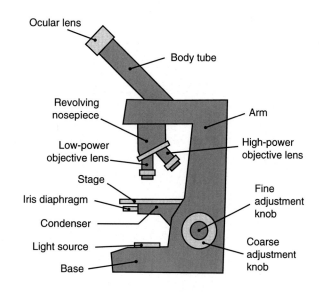

Ocular lens

Body tube

Revolving nosepiece

Arm

Low-power objective lens

High-power objective lens

Stage

Iris diaphragm

Condenser

Light source

Base

Fine adjustment knob

Coarse adjustment knob

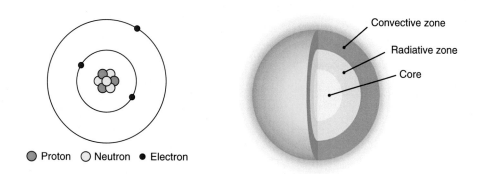

Proton   Neutron   Electron

Convective zone

Radiative zone

Core

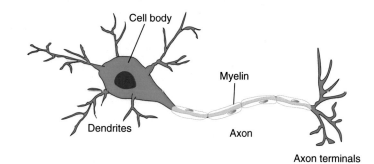

Cell body

Myelin

Dendrites

Axon

Axon terminals

Designing maps

A map shows the spatial arrangement of important features across an area. When designing a map, try to provide a sense of scale so that your audience is better able to perceive physical distances. It is also beneficial to show at least one landmark for orientation, but be careful about including too many landmarks as they may overwhelm the diagram. For example, if creating a geographical map, include the location of a few geographic landmarks, but don't overwhelm the map with locations that aren't important. Also consider adding a "zoomed out" view of a map so that your audience can visualize the region in your map at a global scale.

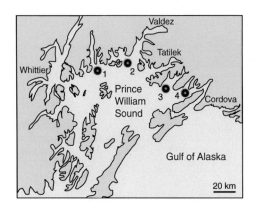

This map of Prince William Sound shows the location of sampling sites for a fisheries study. Note how you automatically assume the blue represents water and the green represents land. There are few geographical landmarks presented, only enough to provide orientation.

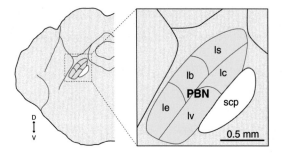

Maps can be of much more than just geological landforms. This map of the mouse brain highlights the location of the parabrachial nucleus. The diagram on the left provides orientation using an illustration of a brain section at low magnification. Color is used to highlight the salient structures and the structure labeled "scp" is used as a landmark for scientists in the field.

Designing sequence maps

Sequence maps visually display sequences of information, such as biological sequences (e.g., DNA, RNA, amino acids) or computational code.

Sequence maps are useful as both research tools and as presentation tools. As a research tool, include as much information as is helpful to further your own goals; however, as a presentation tool, remember to only include as much information as will help your audience understand important aspects of the sequences.

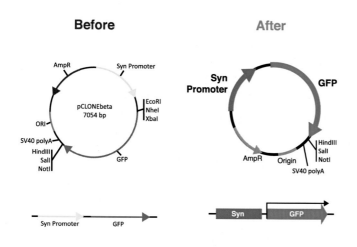

The default settings on most sequence mapping programs are optimized to provide useful information for the user as a research tool, not a presentation tool. Therefore, when presenting a sequence map in a presentation, you may have to enlarge fonts and/or arrows of the structures you want to emphasize, as well minimize or omit information that isn't important. If part of a sequence codes for a color, such as green fluorescent protein (GFP), ensure the sequence is actually represented by that color.

Write out sequence information in a non-proportional font (such as Courier) so that the sequences align. Highlight meaningful information within the code so it is easy for the audience to perceive.

Designing circuit diagrams

Circuit diagrams (also called network or systems diagrams) show the connections between elements in a system or process.

Perhaps the most difficult aspect of designing a network diagram is showing clear, simple connections between multiple elements. When there are several structures in a diagram, it can be hard to clearly separate the lines and arrows. You may need to spend some time trying different strategies of placing lines and labels throughout your diagram to determine the simplest method of representing connections.

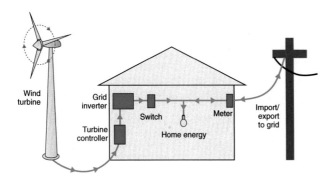

A circuit diagram showing energy pathways to a home connected to a wind turbine and power line.

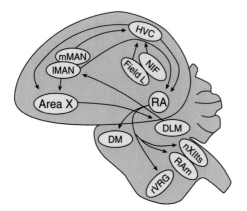

A circuit diagram showing some of the relevant neural populations involved in the process of birds learning to sing superimposed on an avian brain. Crossing lines was avoided as much as possible, but necessary in a couple of locations.

Designing pathway diagrams

Pathway diagrams show how distinct elements interact with each other during a process. Unlike circuit diagrams, pathway diagrams can tell a story with a beginning and end. Action is usually conveyed using arrows.

To make reading a pathway diagram more natural for the audience, order the events in the pathway left to right and top to bottom. Pathways can become extremely complicated very quickly, so be sure to omit elements that don't play an essential role. Finally, emphasize the most important elements with a warmer color than objects that should remain in the background.

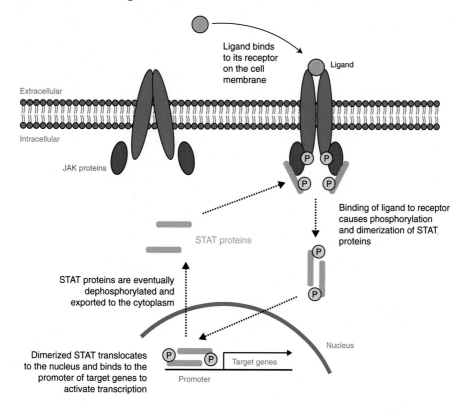

This pathway diagram tells a story of a series of biochemical events in a single illustration. The story starts reading left to right and then top to bottom (before circling back to the top). Foreground elements are in warmer, brighter colors. Explanatory text is in a slightly larger font size than the other labels. While there are many more components to this pathway, only the essential elements are included for clarity. If this figure is intended for a slide presentation, further explanatory power could come from simple animation techniques.

Designing procedural diagrams

A procedural diagram explains a process as a series of discrete steps. These diagrams are useful for helping an audience to understand each stage of an experimental protocol or procedure.

A good way to design a procedural diagram is to start by clearly defining each step in the process before composing any visual elements. Omit steps that aren't important. Express each step as words before adding any accompanying illustrations so that it is easier to only illustrate what is important to show.

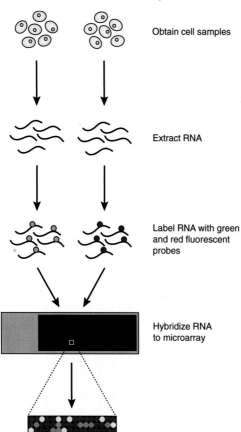

Obtain cell samples

Extract RNA

Label RNA with green and red fluorescent probes

Hybridize RNA to microarray

Analyze hybridization data with computer software. Double-labelled samples will appear yellow.

This procedural diagram describes the process of performing a comparative hybridization experiment using a microarray. The individual steps could be numbered, but numbering is not necessary here because the flow of information is obvious. Many additional steps were deliberately excluded from the diagram (for example, the details involved in extracting RNA) because they distracted from the main focus on microarrays. The colors of the cells were muted because they are not as important as the fluorescent labeling and hybridization data.

Summary: Design principles for diagrams

- Use a diagram in a science presentation when it is more effective or expeditious to visually communicate information compared to using words alone.

- Well-designed diagrams don't have to be highly artistic or seem like they were created by a professional graphic designer. An effective diagram clearly communicates information, and can do so with basic shapes, lines, arrows, and simple labels.

- The best way to start composing a diagram is to define its purpose. It's always a good idea to compose a diagram after stating, "I want my audience to understand that ..."

- Use visual design strategies to emphasize the relative importance of visual elements within a diagram, as well as the importance of the relationships between those elements. Also use design strategies to compose an intuitive order of information within your diagrams.

- Labels within diagrams should be secondary to the visual elements themselves. Ideally they shouldn't add distraction or clutter.

- There are many diagrams commonly used in scientific presentations, including Venn diagrams, flowcharts, tree diagrams, timelines, pictorial diagrams, maps, sequence maps, circuit diagrams, pathway diagrams, and procedural diagrams. Each type of diagram has unique needs and design strategies that can be optimized for maximal communication.

9

Photographs

Photographs instantly communicate data, evidence, ideas, moods, and emotions to an audience. They can quickly present the subject of your experiments to audience members who may be unfamiliar. They can also seize your audience's attention, helping them to understand and remember your content much better than words, bullet points, or graphs alone. Therefore, it is worth the investment in time to learn how to design and edit clear, professional photographs to use in science presentations.

Designing Science Presentations. https://doi.org/10.1016/B978-0-12-815377-2.00009-3

Why show a photo?

Photographs are typically used in science presentations for three reasons:

Photos are great for showing examples of research subjects and experimental paradigms that convey information that cannot be easily expressed in words.

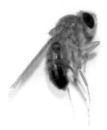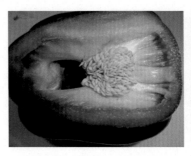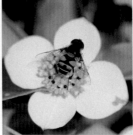

Photos show qualitative data. For example, histological images show data about tissue specimens. Gels and blots from molecular experiments show evidence about gene and protein expression.

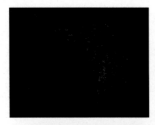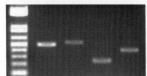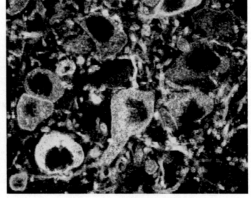

Photos are also excellent visual tools (especially in slide presentations) to communicate ideas and emotions to audience to enhance the context of a scientific story.

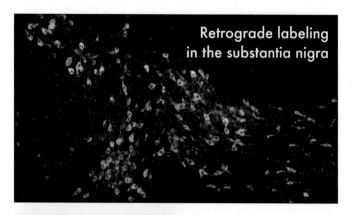

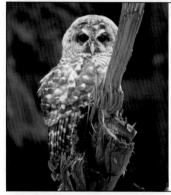

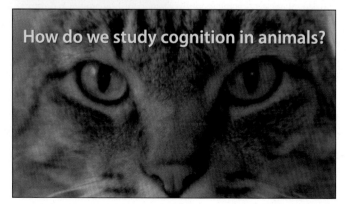

Assume that representative photographic data will be harshly judged

Some of the photographic data that scientists show in presentations are "representative"—a single example of a specimen, histological figure, blot, DNA gel, etc., that serves as an example of what all the other data look like. However, for obvious reasons, most scientists select what they consider their best photographs to show to others. Therefore, a good, critical scientist reviewing representative photographic data should assume that the other data not shown are of *an equal or lesser* quality than the images shown. If the image is suboptimal or difficult to interpret, critical scientists will question the validity of the results of the entire experiment.

Assume that the images you present will be harshly judged based on what you claim. Don't show photographic data unless the results are obvious, clear, and indisputable.

A good way to test the strength of photographic evidence is to show your examples to people unfamiliar with your work, asking what conclusions they would draw from the pictures alone. If they can't immediately tell you the results you intend, your images may not be the most optimal for presentation purposes.

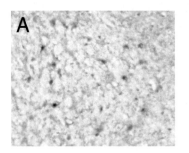 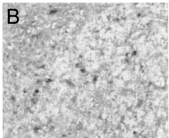

The author of these photomicrographs stained for one protein in brown and another in black and counted the number of cells that express both. He claims that there are approximately three times as many double-labeled cells in Figure A than Figure B. Do you believe him?

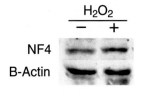

The author of this protein immunoblot claims that H_2O_2 causes a three-fold increase in signal (a darker blot) for NF4. Do you agree?

Be picky about composing and finding images

Many scientists either take their own photos, or find images for slide presentations using internet search engines. Google Images, iStockphoto, Shutterstock, and other image sites are a terrific resource, but make sure that the pictures you choose are the most optimal for your needs. Don't settle on the first images you find, and edit photos as seriously as you would edit text.

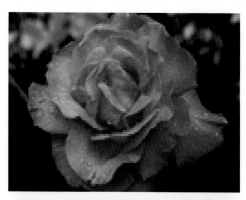

Don't use images that have too low a resolution for your presentation format.

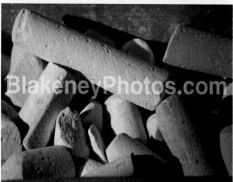

Don't use images that have obvious and distracting watermarks.

Don't use images with suboptimal settings (too light, too dark, too blurry, etc.).

Crop photos to emphasize what is most important

The images you take or find online can often be improved with simple cropping. This technique allows you to frame your images to better suit your needs, focusing on what is most meaningful to you and your narrative.

Original photograph

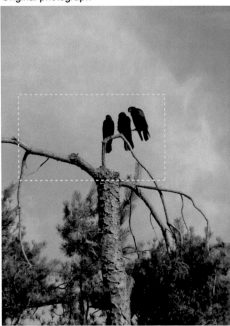

After cropping

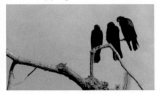

Final presentation slide

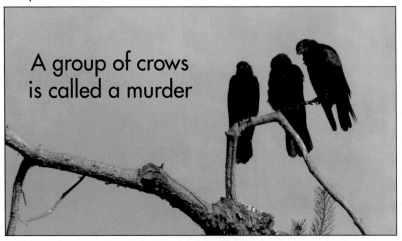

Frame your content using the "rule of thirds"

When cropping images or taking photographs from scratch, consider a fundamental technique used by professional photographers, filmmakers, and graphic designers to make photographs appear more lively and professional: the "rule of thirds."

To use the rule of thirds, imagine a 3 × 3 grid overlaying your field of view and place important elements either along the lines or at the intersections. Arranging meaningful elements in this way will make the subjects of your photographs seem more active and "in the moment" compared with simply placing your subject of interest in the center of the frame. Additionally, studies have shown that people's eyes normally gaze along these intersection points rather than the center of a visual scene.

The rule of thirds grid

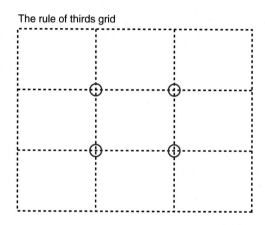

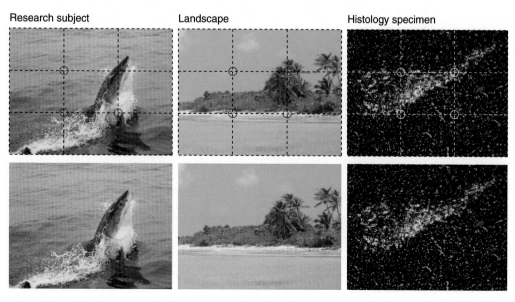

Research subject

Landscape

Histology specimen

Adjust image settings to your needs

Many photograph editing applications allow you to adjust parameters of your images, such as the brightness, contrast, hue, saturation, and sharpness. While these abilities were once limited to photography applications like Photoshop, current versions of word processing applications (Word, Pages) or presentation applications (PowerPoint, Keynote) also allow you to adjust these settings.

There are many reasons you may want to adjust an image—to emphasize certain features, to change the mood or tone, or to better contrast your foregrounds and backgrounds.

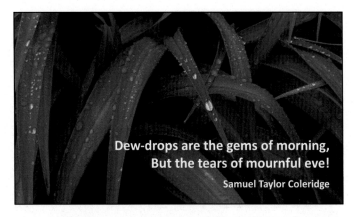

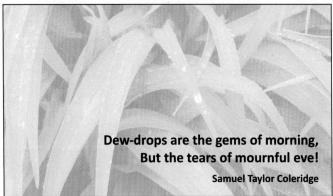

Darkening or lightening a photograph will enhance contrast with the color of the text. Either of these slides would look nice in a slide show. Which version you choose might depend on other factors, for example, the relative brightness of the backgrounds of your other slides.

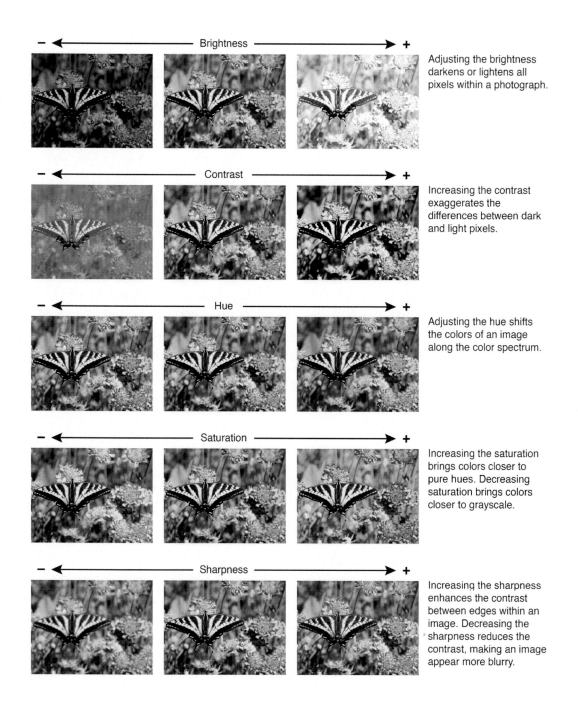

Brightness − → +

Adjusting the brightness darkens or lightens all pixels within a photograph.

Contrast − → +

Increasing the contrast exaggerates the differences between dark and light pixels.

Hue − → +

Adjusting the hue shifts the colors of an image along the color spectrum.

Saturation − → +

Increasing the saturation brings colors closer to pure hues. Decreasing saturation brings colors closer to grayscale.

Sharpness − → +

Increasing the sharpness enhances the contrast between edges within an image. Decreasing the sharpness reduces the contrast, making an image appear more blurry.

Adjust data images *ethically*

There is a very fine line between enhancing an image for optimal quality and manipulating data. While you may have honorable intentions in adjusting an image to make it more clear and professional, be very careful to follow certain guidelines so that you do not risk misrepresenting your results.

General guidelines:

- No specific feature within an image should be enhanced, obscured, moved, removed, or introduced. For example, never erase any part of an image, even if you consider it a smudge or artifact.

- Any modification you do to one image, you must do to any corresponding images. For example, if you modify a picture of an experimental histological specimen (for example, increase brightness or contrasts), you must modify the picture of a control histological specimen in exactly the same way.

- Never combine images from separate microscopy fields of view into a single, merged micrograph unless you make it very clear that you are doing so. Scientists assume that a single image represents a single photograph unless told otherwise.

- In a primary research paper or poster, describe any image enhancements you make to your audience, either in the methods section or figure legends.

- In general, if you feel you are doing something that is crossing an ethical line, don't do it.

Original photo

Unethically enhanced photo

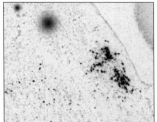 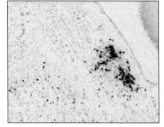

The photograph on the left had some unfortunate artifacts in the upper left corner that the author decided to remove. Although digitally eliminating the artifacts probably did not change the conclusion of the experiment, such an action is unethical. Photographs that present the results of experiments are *data*.

For a more extensive guide on the proper handling of digital photographic data, see an excellent article by Mike Rossner and Kenneth Yamada, "What's in a Picture? The Temptation of Image Manipulation," in *The NIH Catalyst* (May/June 2004) and republished in *The Journal of Cell Biology* (2004, Vol.166(1): 11–15). Although originally intended for biologists, the principles outlined in this guide are applicable to all scientists.

Ensure that labels are secondary to content

When labeling a photographic image, make sure not to distract from the scientific content. Let the data in your image be the main focus and ensure that symbols, arrows, and scale bars play a subtle, supporting role.

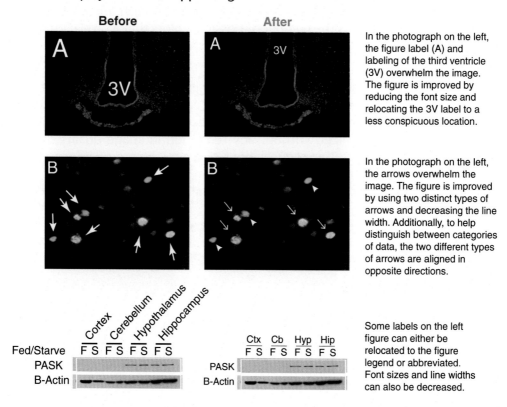

In the photograph on the left, the figure label (A) and labeling of the third ventricle (3V) overwhelm the image. The figure is improved by reducing the font size and relocating the 3V label to a less conspicuous location.

In the photograph on the left, the arrows overwhelm the image. The figure is improved by using two distinct types of arrows and decreasing the line width. Additionally, to help distinguish between categories of data, the two different types of arrows are aligned in opposite directions.

Some labels on the left figure can either be relocated to the figure legend or abbreviated. Font sizes and line widths can also be decreased.

The differences between image file formats

Digital images are stored and recognized by software applications in various file formats, including JPEGs, TIFFs, GIFs, and PNGs. All of these formats code for pixels, with each pixel containing values for color and brightness. The file size of an image (measured in bytes—there are 8 bits in every byte) increases with the number of pixels composing an image, as well as the number of possible colors that a pixel can represent. An 8-bit pixel (1 byte) stores 256 colors, while a 24-bit pixel (3 bytes) stores 16 million colors.

The goal of various image file formats is to code for images using the smallest file size possible. To accomplish this goal, the images are "compressed" using algorithms. In general, there are two major categories of compression. In a **lossless compression** format, the file size is minimized without any reduction in image quality. In a **lossy compression** format, an algorithm reduces the file size by discarding information that is likely to be invisible to the human eye. Most of these algorithms have a variable quality threshold—as compression increases, the quality of an image decreases.

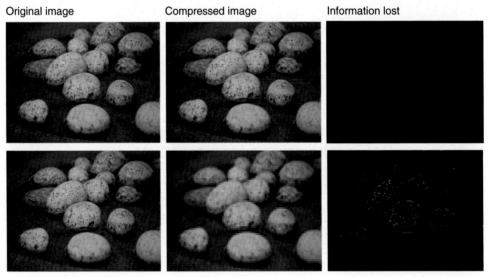

Examples of lossy image compression. The top row shows an ideal compression: the information that is lost is invisible to the human eye. As the level of compression increases, as in the bottom row, the discarded information becomes noticable.

The following four file formats are the most common:

JPEG   **Joint Photographic Experts Group format.** JPEGs store information as 8 bits per color (red, green, and blue) for a 24-bit total. This format uses lossy compression, which usually isn't noticeable unless the compression level is relatively high. JPEGs usually have a relatively smaller file size than PNGs and especially TIFFs, so they are a great format for sending and receiving (which is why they are often the default format for encoding photographs in most smartphones and digital cameras).

TIFF   **Tagged Image File Format.** TIFFs save 8 bits or 16 bits per color (red, green, and blue) for 24-bit and 48-bit totals. TIFFs can utilize either lossy or lossless compression, depending on the software reading the format. When printing high-resolution images, it is recommended that you use the TIFF format because of the lossless compression. Therefore, TIFF may be the best file format choice when designing written and poster presentations—in fact, many scientific journals require figures to be produced in the TIFF format instead of JPEGs. The major drawback of TIFF images is that they usually have larger file sizes compared to other formats, which make them less optimal for slide shows, websites, and sharing images with others.

GIF   **Graphics Interchange Format.** GIFs store information at 8 bits per pixel, reducing the colors in an image to just 256. Therefore, GIFs are usually smaller in file size but also a poor choice for storing detailed graphics and photographs. They feature lossless compression, but their overall image quality is usually relatively poorer than JPEGs or TIFFs. The advantage to using the GIF format is that it is possible to store multiple images within a single file, allowing for simple animations that last a few seconds. Therefore, the main use of GIFs are in downloadable animations, logos, and clip art.

PNG   **Portable Network Graphics Format.** The PNG format was intentionally created for small file sizes in websites and other media. Unlike GIFs, which are 8-bit and limited to 256 colors, PNG images are 24-bit and can therefore specify 16 million colors. Like GIFs, PNGs feature lossless compression.

Ideal image resolutions for different presentation formats

In general, it is always best to use high-resolution images in your presentations. However, as resolution increases, so does file size, and even the newest, faster computers can show a decrease in performance when opening and manipulating documents with multiple high-resolution images. The best way to optimize the balance between resolution and file size is to maximize the resolution of your images to the point at which the eye can no longer detect any increase in quality. Increasing resolution beyond this point will increase file size without a corresponding increase in perceived image quality.

When saving images for your presentations, you can choose to save at different resolutions by changing the pixels-per-inch (ppi) settings.

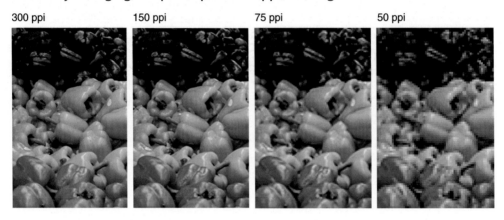

Each presentation format requires different resolutions:

Written presentation: For images that will appear in published journals, photographs should be submitted at 300 pixels per inch (ppi). Line drawings need to be even higher resolution—typically around 600 ppi, so the lines and shapes appear as crisp as possible. Although research articles and review articles are typically printed, many readers view them as PDFs which can be magnified on a screen. Therefore, written presentations typically have the highest resolution requirements.

Slide presentation: Slide presentations typically do not have the same high-resolution image requirements as printed presentations. A standard slide size is 1024 × 768 pixels while a widescreen slide is typically 1920 × 1080 pixels. Because most computers and projectors now use high definition displays, 300 ppi is optimal for most photographs.

Poster presentation: Posters should be printed at 150–300 ppi. 300 ppi is the professional standard, used by professional marketing agencies for advertisements and banners. However, in most cases, readers won't be able to tell the difference between 150 and 300 ppi.

Summary: Design principles for photographs

- Photographs are great for showing pictures of your research specimens and experimental set-up, for presenting qualitative data, or (in slide presentations) for bringing your content to life.

- Ensure that the images you present in your science presentations are of the highest quality. When a scientist presents a photo as a "representative image," it is actually probably one of the most convincing images. Therefore, ensure that your images are so good that your subsequent conclusions are obvious and credible.

- Be picky about the images you present, rejecting images with suboptimal resolution, brightness, contrast, etc., or images that have distracting logos or watermarks.

- Consider cropping your photos to emphasize what is most important.

- If you take or crop a photograph, consider using the "rule of thirds" to frame your subject in a way that makes your photograph seem more active and visually compelling.

- Adjust photographic parameters such as brightness, contrast, hue, saturation, and sharpness to ensure your photos are as clear and sharp as possible.

- When adjusting photographs that present data, make sure you do so in a way that is ethical and that does not create artificial distinctions between different datasets.

- When you apply labels to photographs, do so in a way that ensures that labels are secondary to the content itself.

- Save your photographs in the most appropriate file format (JPEG, TIFF, GIF, PNG) that preserves details while optimizing file sizes.

- Save your photographs at the appropriate resolution for your presentation format to show the best images possible at the lowest file size.

Part 3

**Expressing scientific ideas
in written presentations**

10

Research articles

A scientist's success is primarily measured by the quantity and quality of their peer-reviewed research articles. To publish regularly, scientists must have both great scientific content and the skills necessary to accurately present this content in written form. When poorly written, journal editors and anonymous reviewers are less enthusiastic about manuscripts, especially if they cannot adequately understand the study. When well written, a paper presents research in the best possible light and increases the chances that a manuscript will be accepted. Fortunately, all scientists can develop as writers, and there are proven strategies for optimizing the various sections of a research article.

Designing Science Presentations. https://doi.org/10.1016/B978-0-12-815377-2.00010-X

The purpose of a research article

The most important reason to publish a research article is to add your results to the permanent domain of scientific knowledge—the scientific record. Unlike a slide presentation or poster presentation, the work published in a research article is enduring and immutable. Your published work is always available for anyone to access—now, 20 years from now, perhaps even hundreds of years from now.

Research articles represent the ultimate, final product of a scientific study. A published paper shows that you have completed a research project, from beginning to end, and the peer-reviewed results are indefinitely available for anyone in the world to access.

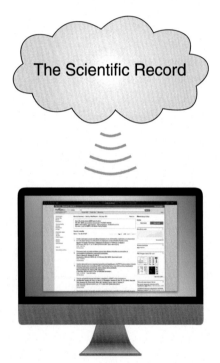

The Scientific Record

In the modern scientific era, the scientific record exists digitally in the cloud. Most scholarly articles from the past are available online, and every article published now and in the future will be available online. To publish a research article means to permanently add your science to the scientific record such that it can be theoretically accessed by anyone, anywhere, anytime.

Of course, there are many other important reasons to publish research articles. Publishing papers establishes your reputation among your peers and demonstrates to your funding agencies that you are a responsible grantee who delivers results. Graduate students need papers to get good postdoctoral fellowships, postdocs need papers to get good permanent jobs, and principal investigators need papers to get funding and promotions. Therefore, writing and publishing strong research articles is one of the most important skills a scientist must learn.

The structure of a research article

The structure of a research article depends on the specific formatting guidelines of the scientific journal to which you submit your work. Most journals use subheadings with dedicated introduction, results, and discussion sections. Some journals do not employ subheadings at all, and read as one continuous article. In either case, a well-written research article will usually contain the following sections:

Title: A specific statement that conveys the topic and conclusion of the paper.

Abstract: A complete summary of the paper.

Introduction: The beginning of a paper that transitions from a general background to a specific research question or goal.

Materials and Methods: A brief but detailed description about the tools and methods you used to perform experiments and analyze results.

Results: A presentation of all of your experiments and data, represented both as text and in tables, graphs, diagrams, and photographs.

Discussion: An opportunity to discuss your interpretation of your results and explore your findings within the context of the larger scientific record.

References: Your citations.

Supplemental Materials: Additional figures, videos, and sometimes elaboration of methods and computational analyses that will appear online only.

Depending on the journal and category of article, these sections will be of different lengths or appear in a different order. For example, some journals place the materials and methods section just after the introduction, others place it at the end of the paper. Some even place this section entirely online in a supplemental methods section.

The title should emphasize what is most important

The title of your research article is the most important factor in determining whether your article will be read at all. Hundreds or thousands of scientists will come across your title in a searchable online database, and their impression of your title will determine whether they want to read your abstract or entire paper. Therefore, your title should emphasize what is most important and exciting about your research project. Because titles usually have a word limit, every single word counts.

The best titles are often conclusions because they communicate the most information to your audience.

Before	The effect of positive reinforcement on mathematics performance in 10-year-old females
After	Positive reinforcement increases mathematics performance in 10-year-old females
Before	The role of Sufl2 in primary necrosis
After	Sufl2 blocks primary necrosis by preventing mitochondrial outer membrane permeabilization
Before	Gene expression profiles of inner and outer hair cells
After	Comparative gene expression profiles of inner and outer hair cells reveals a multitude of uniquely expressed genes

Sometimes authors like to emphasize methods in their titles—e.g., "fMRI analysis of visual attention." You must decide what it is that you want to emphasize and what will be most informative to readers, however, methods are almost always secondary to larger conclusions. Exciting methods come and go, but conclusions are always interesting.

Methods-based	Optogenetic investigation of the inferior colliculus in echolocating bats
Conclusion-based	The inferior colliculus is tonotopically organized in echolocating bats

Effective abstracts tell a complete story

Most people who come across your paper in a journal or search engine will decide whether to read your full paper based on your abstract. In fact, in online search engines, your abstract is likely to be the only part of your paper that your audience will see at first. If they want to keep reading, they will have to actively access your paper. Therefore, your abstract must be well written. If it is difficult to read or is not forthcoming with information, it will potentially turn away readers.

A good abstract is like a miniature version of your entire paper, with a background, scientific question, results, interpretation, and discussion, all within a single paragraph.

The structure of an abstract:

Pacific salmon hatcheries raise and release juvenile fish to supplement wild stocks and enhance commercial harvest. Over 100 salmon hatcheries in Hokkaido, Japan, raise and release a total of over one billion chum salmon fry each year to supplement wild populations that have decreased steadily since the 1930s. Whether sufficient prey are available to absorb the additional consumption demand by hatchery-produced chum salmon is unknown. The increased abundance of juveniles from hatchery production has elicited concerns that the carrying capacity for juvenile chum salmon has been reached or exceeded; juvenile chum salmon could potentially become food-limited at one or more stages in their life cycle in one or more geographic regions. Here we show that the localized standing stock biomass of key prey was not enough to sustain the high level of consumption required by chum salmon to satisfy observed growth during the first five months at sea. The high percentage of prey biomass consumed and the fact that growth and consumption rates were higher for all cohorts during years of high survival indicate that Hokkaido chum salmon are food limited during the juvenile stage. Competition for limited prey resources between hatchery and wild salmon could present potential risks to the health of wild stocks in particular. Our findings demonstrate that the potential benefits of hatchery programs should be weighed against risks to wild stocks and the greater ecosystem. Furthermore, production should be aligned with the carrying capacity of the region.

- 1-2 sentences to introduce the paper to any scientist
- 2-3 sentences to introduce the paper to more specialized scientists within your field
- 1-2 sentences to describe the main findings
- 2-3 sentences to elaborate on what was observed
- 1-2 sentences about the conclusions and implications of the study

Searchable online databases often include all of the words in the abstract in the search queries. Therefore, if someone types a word that is found in your abstract into a search field, your paper will be listed in the search results. Therefore, be strategic about including words in your abstract that will help your paper reach a larger audience.

Effective introductions lead to a specific research goal

The introduction to a research article begins broadly, introducing readers to the current state of a field. Throughout a series of paragraphs (depending on the guidelines of the journal), the introduction then narrows in scope to lead to a specific research goal or hypothesis. Therefore, an effective introduction has four crucial goals:

(1) To declare the overall topic for the reader (e.g., dark matter, obesity, seed dispersal, chemical synthesis)

(2) To provide relevant background material to demonstrate the work leading up to your experiments

(3) To define a clear problem or research question and state why it is important

(4) To clearly define the purpose of the study and how it addresses the open problem

After your audience reads your introduction, they should be able to accurately describe your overall field, the work that preceded your paper, what is unknown, how your paper solved for the unknown, and why it is all important.

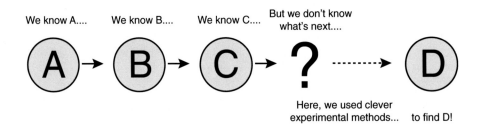

Most of your introduction will consist of a brief literature review. When citing papers in the introduction, be strategic about the papers you cite. The anonymous reviewers who receive your manuscript are likely to work in the same field as you and will appreciate having their work referenced. Therefore, be deliberate about including papers written by labs within your field that are likely to receive your paper for review.

Because much of the introduction is about the current state of scientific knowledge, you should write your introduction in the *present* tense.

Materials and methods sections allow studies to be reproducible

The purpose of a methods section is to provide enough detail about how you conducted your study such that an independent investigator could repeat your exact experiments. To make this section easy to read and to help your audience find information quickly, be sure to use subheadings for each distinct method performed. Don't cite other papers so readers have to look up methods on their own from another source (e.g., "We performed this procedure following the methods of Formas et al."). Instead, provide enough information such that someone could use the same reagents and procedures without having to look anything up from another source.

Make a special effort to describe all of your materials such that others could perform experiments with exactly the same reagents and products that you used.

Details to include about materials:

- The number, age, source, and (for animals) sex of research organisms
- The name and version of all computer software used for data analysis
- The source and product numbers of all non-commonly used chemical reagents
- The source and product numbers of all commercially available antibodies
- The names and sources of any specialized scientific equipment
- The exact genetic locations or sequences used in cloning or subcloning experiments
- The spatial coordinates of any specific locations where samples were collected or a study was performed

In truth, many readers will probably skip your methods section. Depending on your field and the nature of your study, there is a high likelihood that no other scientist will even attempt reproducing your experiments. However, they will want to know exactly how you came to your conclusions and how they could perform the same experiments if necessary. The potential for reproducibility must always exist, even if the likelihood does not.

Aside from reproducibility, a secondary goal of the materials and methods section is to establish your credibility. When the methods section is well written, you come across as knowing what you are doing, and your audience is more likely to trust your results.

Because your experiments took place in the past, you should write your methods section in the *past* tense.

Provide your results section with context

Because science papers can be long and complex, it is extremely helpful to continually remind your readers of the rationale, methodology, and ultimate conclusions of the experiments you perform. Therefore, it is important not to write about experimental results in isolation with no context.

The results section should be written such that each 1–2 paragraphs exists as a "mini-paper," complete with its own rationale, statement of methods, results, and conclusion.

Consider beginning the first or second sentence in each of your paragraphs with the word "To. …" This technique will force you to begin each part of your results section with a justification of why you performed the specific experiments you describe.

Before   We next overexpressed full-length versions of Tav1, Farr3, and Farr6 in HEK293T cells and performed co-immunoprecipitation experiments using an antibody to Tav1. Tav1 interacted with both Farr3 and Farr6.

After   To determine if Tav1 interacts with Farr3 and Farr6, we overexpressed full-length versions of these proteins in HEK293T cells and performed co-immunoprecipitation experiments using an antibody to Tav1. We found that Tav1 interacted with both Farr3 and Farr6, indicating that Tav1 interacts with either receptor *ex vivo*.

Before   Following injections of 4% (hypertonic) or 0.9% (isotonic) saline directly into the OVLT, we stained for Fos, an indirect marker of neural activity. We found a statistically significant increase in Fos expression in the OVLT from mice receiving hypertonic saline ($P < 0.05$, student's t-test).

After   To determine if the OVLT increases activity in response to hypertonicity, we injected 4% (hypertonic) or 0.9% (isotonic) saline directly into the OVLT region, sacrificed the animals, and stained the brain sections for Fos, an indirect marker of neural activity. We found a statistically significant increase in Fos expression in the OVLT from mice receiving hypertonic saline compared to control mice ($P < 0.05$, student's t-test), demonstrating that hypertonicity increases activity in this brain region.

When writing the results, use the *past* tense to describe what you did, and the *present* tense to describe your conclusions and what was learned from the experiment.

Achieve harmony between figures and text

Designing good tables, graphs, diagrams, and photographs was described in Chapters 6–9, respectively. Your figures should ideally communicate information on their own for any reader who wants to quickly understand the main findings of the paper (some scientists read papers by focusing exclusively on your figures).

The best titles of figure legends are conclusions, and the legend itself should convey everything necessary to understand the symbols, lines, and bars in the tables and charts.

Try to avoid describing your figures in the text. Your readers don't want descriptions of figures, they want descriptions of results. Therefore, focus your results section on your experiments and findings, citing your figures as you would cite references.

Before	Fig. 3a shows that nitric acid caused structural degradation of the carbon nanotubes.
After	Nitric acid caused structural degradation of the carbon nanotubes (Fig. 3a).
Before	We present the geographical coordinates used in this study in Table 3.
After	We placed eight atmospheric monitoring stations within a 6-km^2 area (Table 3).
Before	In Fig. 7, we show a diagram depicting an indirect feedback loop between miRNAs and SMB7.
After	Our results suggest a model in which miRNAs indirectly regulate SMB7 (Fig. 7).

Many journals also allow authors to submit supplementary figures and videos that readers can access online. Most readers won't expend the effort to access these figures unless they are particularly interested, so only put information that isn't crucial to the main findings of the paper in your supplementary figures. Usually these figures validate or demonstrate methods rather than contribute novel scientific findings.

Use your discussion section to add reflection and insight

Most scientists find the discussion section the most difficult to write because, unlike the other sections, there is no obvious structure or information to include. In general, this section is your opportunity to briefly summarize your findings, interpret any interesting, contradictory, or confusing results, and place your results in the context of the larger scientific record.

Don't waste your discussion section by restating everything you already described in the introduction and results. Instead, use your discussion to add depth and insight to your results.

Don't use your discussion to …

- Recapitulate all of your results. Feel free to begin your discussion with a brief recap of your results, but don't describe all of them throughout your discussion section. Only discuss those data that require further explanation.

- Write a discussion section that is too long. How long is too long? The length depends on the nature of your field and your findings, but in general, a discussion section should be shorter than your results section.

- Speculate on future directions. In slide or poster presentations, it can be informative to discuss future experiments because those presentation formats usually describe works in progress. Leave them out of papers. They usually come across as too speculative, and sometimes anonymous reviewers will ask why you didn't already do those experiments and include them in your current submission.

- Overstate your conclusions. See the "hierarchy of claims" in Chapter 5.

Instead, use your discussion to …

- Highlight the significance of your results and the contribution of your study to your field.

- Show how your results are in agreement or disagreement with previous studies.

- Discuss any results from your study that seem confusing or paradoxical.

- Consider alternate explanations of your findings.

- Discuss the practical applications of your work.

Additionally, it is always nice to end a paper with a final conclusion that summarizes the major contributions of the paper in one or two sentences and establishes its place within the larger scientific record. This conclusion not only provides your paper with a solid ending but also serves as a final take-home message for your audience.

Avoid common reasons for rejection

When writing a research paper, it can be helpful to think about not only the qualities that will make your manuscript a success, but also the mistakes to avoid. Editors of scientific journals are usually very open and honest about the most common reasons why manuscripts are rejected for publication. Some of these reasons are obviously about the content of a manuscript, but many are actually about the writing of the article itself.

Problems with content

- The results do not justify the conclusions
- The topic of the paper is too specialized for the journal
- Inappropriate experimental design
- Lack of novelty
- The research is trivial or incomplete
- The research is too similar to the author's previous publication(s)
- An important interpretation or explanation of experiments is missing

Problems with writing

- The author did not follow directions regarding how to write the manuscript
- The manuscript is poorly written and hard to understand
- Speculation in the discussion is not based on data and unwarranted
- Improper references cited in the introduction or discussion
- Poorly designed figures
- Too many errors, typos, mistakes

When reviewing and revising your manuscript, think about your paper from the point of view of an editor, and see if you can "reject" it before you even submit. Ask colleagues for harsh feedback, both about your content and about your writing. Consider the lists above and try to avoid the common mistakes made by others.

Summary: Design principles for writing research articles

- Research articles represent the ultimate, final product of a scientific study. You should assume that your published work will be indefinitely available for anyone to access.

- Research articles always consist of a title, abstract, introduction, materials and methods, results, discussion, and references sections, and many include a supplemental materials section. There are strategies for making each section most helpful to the reader.

- Effective titles of research articles communicate the most important aspects of the study and communicate as much information as possible.

- An effective abstract completely summarizes your paper within a single paragraph and highlights why the results are novel.

- An effective introduction highlights the most interesting previous studies in your field and leads to the unknown question that drove your research project forward.

- The materials and methods section provides enough detail such that a study is reproducible without forcing the reader to consult other studies.

- Each 1–2 paragraphs of a results section should come across as its own "mini-paper," complete with its own rationale, statement of methods, results, and conclusion. To ensure that you provide a rationale, consider starting each part of your results section with the word, "To .... "

- Don't refer to your figures or tables within the text ... instead, state the information and then cite the figures and tables, just as you would cite references.

- Use your discussion section to add new insight or understanding to your research article, not just to summarize or repeat the previous sections.

- When writing a research article, keep in mind the common reasons that papers are rejected, both regarding the content and the writing style.

11

Review articles

Writing a review article is completely different from writing a research article or research proposal. Broader in scope, a review is less about your work and more about an entire scientific topic. Furthermore, a review doesn't have an inherent structure—there are no standard sections, figure requirements, or common expectations about how you discuss the literature. The freedom to compose a review with your own vision and ideas can be liberating, but also intimidating—especially if you have never written a review before. Fortunately, there are many useful strategies for approaching the composition of a review so that it is a pleasure to read and adds insight to your field of study.

Designing Science Presentations. https://doi.org/10.1016/B978-0-12-815377-2.00011-1

The purpose of a review article

A review article assembles the results of dozens or even hundreds of primary research articles into a coherent narrative about a specific scientific topic.

One of the major purposes of a review article is to make sense of the scientific literature. When you enter a search term into an online database, the result is often hundreds, if not thousands, of papers that may or may not be relevant to your interests. If you are interested in learning about a new scientific topic, it is difficult to know which papers are the most important to read. A good review article that describes the current state of a field is an invaluable resource.

However, a good review should be much more than just a list of relevant information. If the purpose of a review were only to itemize papers on a single topic, a review could consist entirely of a references section. Instead, a good review provides a comprehensive understanding of a subject. It explains a topic from a bird's-eye view of the literature, arranging ideas into a larger narrative. When writing a review, you need to think about not only what material you present, but also *how* you present it.

The best reviews compare and contrast different studies and offer opinions on the relative strength and importance of ideas. They also add something new: a scientific model, a new insight, or a suggestion for how a field can move forward to solve a scientific problem.

The audience of a review is usually much broader than that of a primary research paper. Your readers will consist of scientists in the field, but also other scientists who want to learn about a new topic. Therefore, your review needs to be both specific enough to satisfy colleagues in your field and broad enough to inform novices from a different scientific background.

Designing Science Presentations

When writing a review, you start with the chaos that is the scientific literature...

...you identify the research articles that are the most important and salient to your topic...

...and you analyze different categories of information to provide meaningful conclusions about your topic. In the end, you make a statement about a scientific topic that is greater than the sum of its parts.

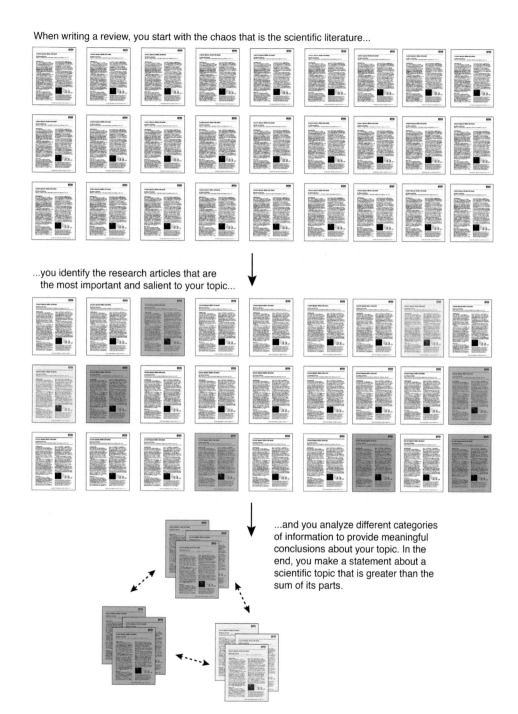

Choose a way to make sense of the literature

Before you begin writing a review, be clear about the way in which you want to present and discuss scientific ideas. Consider that you can present information about your topic with varying degrees of insight, and more insightful reviews have a greater impact on a scientific field. The different degrees of insight range from simply explaining other studies to constructing new ideas based on a synthesis of the information.

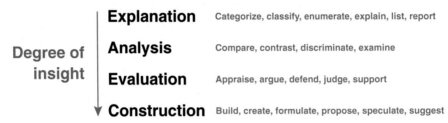

Explanation: Provides a summary of the primary literature. It is the simplest way to present information in a review and usually most beneficial to readers new to your topic.

- Surveys all of the recent publications that describe a single phenomenon, subject, or technique
- Describes how a natural phenomenon or complicated technique works

Analysis: Compares and contrasts multiple studies.

- Compares the relative advantages and disadvantages of an experimental strategy in the study of a particular phenomenon
- Examines how a phenomenon in one species exhibits differences compared with a phenomenon in a different species
- Discriminates between the experimental designs of two studies that produced contrasting results

Evaluation: Judges the quality of primary papers and forms an opinion.

- Determines the conclusions of a series of studies to be inaccurate
- Argues in favor of a scientific theory
- Defends an unpopular scientific point of view

Construction: Offers new ideas that add depth and insight to a field. Truly original concepts in a review may impact a field even more than an original research study.

- Proposes a scientific model based on the results of several studies
- Speculates on a new way to accomplish a goal
- Proposes an experimental strategy to answer an unresolved question

Strategies to improve the readability of your review

Review articles are unlike other forms of scientific writing in that they have no inherent structure. Unlike research papers and proposals, there is no set specification for the quantity or types of subsections found in the main text. There is also no requirement to include figures or tables. Therefore, when someone begins reading a review, they typically have no idea what to expect other than a vague notion of the subject matter. As the author, you can help your readers by providing an overall sense of structure and readability.

Design a review article to maximize the reading experience of your audience, considering not only the subject matter you present, but also how you present it.

Include subdivisions throughout your paper to provide organization and structure. Unless your review is relatively short, your main text will be too long to flow undivided. Because you don't have natural subheadings as you would in a research paper (e.g., methods, results, discussion) include your own subheadings that clearly follow a logical narrative.

Explicitly outline your review in the abstract and/or introduction. To help your audience immediately perceive the overall objective and structure of your review, deliberately introduce readers to the structure in the very beginning (e.g., "In this review, we will first ..., next we will ..., finally we will ...."). Readers will appreciate a roadmap of where the review will eventually take them so they know what to expect.

Include as many informative figures and tables as possible. Figures and tables are always necessary in research papers, slide presentations, and posters, but they aren't explicitly required in reviews. That doesn't mean you shouldn't include them—quite the contrary. Diagrams that illustrate concepts or tables that categorize primary papers help communicate messages and make your paper more visually interesting. In fact, the more visually stimulating a review appears, the more likely potential readers are to actually read from start to finish.

Choose and highlight the best references. Many scientists read reviews primarily to gain an understanding of the most salient primary papers in a field. Help your readers by showing them which papers are potentially the most interesting. Some journals allow (or require) annotated references in which you highlight some papers as particularly interesting. You can also highlight references by designing a table that presents categories of information and the references in which readers can find out more about them. Finally, in the text, be sure to highlight your favorite reviews with descriptive statements that add value (e.g., "A transformative study from Cross et al. showed that ....").

Writing a review article from scratch

When you begin composing a research paper or proposal, it is often possible to write certain sections (such as your methods) relatively easily because you are personally familiar with the subject matter and probably already have an idea about what you want to communicate. In contrast, when writing a review, you shouldn't attempt writing anything until you have thoroughly outlined how you want to present your information.

The following strategy seems to work well for many scientists:

1. **Identify the specific topic of your review.** Examine the literature to determine if a quality review about the same topic already exists. If so, consider slightly adjusting your focus so that your review doesn't reinvent someone else's work and will have a greater impact on your field.

2. **Search the literature for all relevant papers.** Surveying the literature can be daunting, and don't be intimidated if your first few searches using internet databases return thousands of results. Try increasing the specificity of your searches using a variety of search terms. It may also help to narrow your results by only examining papers from the past few years, which will probably cite the important older papers, anyway. Also consider only examining papers from the highest impact journals in your field so that the papers are likely to carry more transformative results.

3. **Once you have performed an initial search, try not to become focused on other review articles.** One can become crazy by continually evaluating how other authors addressed your topic, even if your focus is slightly different.

4. **As you read papers, separate them into useful groups.** Some people like to use a spreadsheet to categorize papers; others put papers into different piles on their desk. Do whatever works best for you to categorize and keep track of information.

5. **Consider the level of insight you would like to provide your readers.** Are you explaining and listing concepts, or are you also analyzing, evaluating, and offering opinions of your own?

6. **Create a rough outline or skeleton of your review.** Creating an outline is probably the single most important aspect of the writing process because you begin making important decisions about the structure, scope, and depth of your review. Decide not only what information you will present, but what info you will *not* include.

7. **Think about useful diagrams and tables you can provide your readers.** Especially consider when a diagram is more explanatory than a section of text.

8. **When you write your first draft, start with major headings and concepts instead of specific references.** If you start the writing process by focusing on structure, all of your details will fall into place when you add them later.

Summary: Design principles for writing review articles

- A review article synthesizes dozens of primary research articles into a comprehensive narrative about a field of knowledge.

- Review articles can synthesize the scientific literature in different ways. They can be explanative, providing a summary of recent articles; they can offer analysis, comparing and contrasting scientific studies; they can be evaluative, appraising studies and supporting points of view; or they can be constructive, offering new points of view. Before writing an article, determine what level of analysis you want your review to offer.

- Help your readers appreciate the structure of your review article by including subdivisions throughout the review article and outlining these subdivisions in your abstract and/or introduction.

- Include as many informative figures and tables as possible to visually convey and synthesize information.

- Choose and highlight the best references to help your readers learn the best sources of primary information.

12

Research proposals

Writing research proposals is such a common task among scientists that sometimes we forget what we are literally doing: asking for a substantial sum of money. Ask yourself, what would it take for you to give someone the amount of money you are requesting? What would you want to know about the person asking for hundreds of thousands of dollars and how they planned to use it? Although research proposals discuss scientific ideas, they are ultimately about convincing an organization that your objectives are worth the time, effort, budget, and other support that you request.

Designing Science Presentations. https://doi.org/10.1016/B978-0-12-815377-2.00012-3

The purpose of a research proposal: to justify

The obvious goal of a research proposal is to obtain funding for your experiments, your salary, and (at the faculty level) your personnel. If you are an undergraduate or graduate student, you may write research proposals for class assignments or your qualifying exam, but the main function of these exercises is to prepare you for writing a real grant or fellowship proposal in the future.

To achieve your goal of securing funding, it is useful to think of your proposal as having a fundamental purpose: to justify.

The ultimate goal of a research proposal is to justify why an outside organization should give you financial support instead of someone else.

Your research proposal may be well written and your scientific ideas may seem obvious to you, but if you don't clearly justify your rationale and thought process, your proposal will fail to convince your readers that your ideas are original, important, logical and feasible.

What you must justify in a research proposal:

- Your scientific topic is important
- Your specific scientific question/goal is important
- You are an expert on your topic and have a command of the relevant scientific literature
- You are fully qualified to perform the study
- Your institution is a terrific place to perform the study
- Your preliminary experiments suggest a likely chance of success
- Your experimental design is logical
- Your methods are feasible and you have the necessary expertise to perform them
- You have alternative approaches in case your plan is initially unsuccessful
- The results of your study will make a substantial contribution to a scientific field

Writing a research proposal requires a different kind of salesmanship than other forms of scientific writing. If you are new to the process, it is highly beneficial to enroll in a grant-writing workshop at your institution and examine several previously funded proposals. Notice how these successful proposals justify nearly everything they describe.

Pleasing your reviewers

Different funding organizations review research proposals in different ways. Your proposal will typically be considered by one or two primary reviewers and possibly a third who may offer additional opinions when necessary. Your proposal will probably be discussed within a larger group of reviewers, although only those assigned to your proposal will read it thoroughly.

Always consult the funding organization's instructions to determine how reviewers will evaluate your proposal. Every grant or fellowship has different criteria, but the following are typical:

Significance. Does the proposal address an important problem or a critical barrier to progress in the field?

Investigator. Are the principal investigator [this term also refers to graduate students and postdocs applying for fellowships] and other collaborators well-suited to the project? If in the early stages of a career, do they have appropriate experience and training? If established, have they demonstrated an ongoing record of accomplishments that have advanced their fields?

Innovation. Does the application challenge and seek to shift current research or clinical practice paradigms by utilizing novel theoretical concepts, approaches or methodologies, instrumentation, or interventions?

Approach. Are the overall strategy, methodology, and analyses well-reasoned and appropriate to accomplish the specific aims of the project? Are potential problems, alternative strategies, and benchmarks for success presented?

Environment. Will the scientific environment where the work will be performed contribute to the probability of success? Will the project benefit from unique features of the scientific environment, subject populations, or collaborative arrangements?

After reading your proposal, the answers to all of the above questions must be an enthusiastic YES.

In addition to the above criteria, funding agencies will require detailed information about your personal background, physical setting, use of humans or vertebrate animals, etc.

Reviewers will also expect a professional, well-written proposal. Because only a small percentage of applications are likely to be funded, every detail counts. Reviewers will ensure that you followed all directions and will care that your writing is accurate in grammar and style. Good writing implies good science.

The structure of a research proposal

Every funding agency has its own guidelines for the different sections of a grant or fellowship, and you absolutely must read and follow the instructions to ensure you write your proposal correctly. Usually a research proposal contains the following sections:

Title. A succinct, one-sentence description of your research proposal.

Executive Summary (also called the Abstract or Specific Aims). This introductory text is a half-page or one-page summary of your entire research proposal in which you present your entire rationale, purpose, and specific aims. If well written, reviewers will look forward to reading the rest of your proposal. However, if you do not convey a clear sense of importance and novelty, some funding agencies may decide that your proposal is inadequate based on this section alone.

Background and Significance. This section consists of a brief literature review in which you clearly describe the relevant past work on your topic, leading to a declaration of your hypothesis or goal. If the work you cite does not relate to the research you propose, your reviewers will doubt your rationale (not to mention your scholarship) and your proposal will not be funded.

Preliminary Data. Some funding agencies will require that you present preliminary data. This section demonstrates that you have initial success toward achieving your goal, increasing the likelihood that your proposed experiments will lead to positive results.

Research Design and Methods. The meat of your proposal, this section contains a complete description of your research plan, usually divided into two or three individual specific aims. For each specific aim, you should address the following topics (even if not explicitly required by your funding agency):

    Rationale. The purpose of the experiments.

    Experimental Design. The experiments you will perform and the methods you will use to answer your scientific question.

    Potential results and interpretations. All of the potential outcomes of your experiments, and how you will interpret each.

    Potential problems and alternative approaches. The experimental or technical problems that can cause your experiment to fail, as well as your alternative plans to ensure your study can continue.

Conclusion. A brief paragraph to cement why your proposal is highly important to fund.

Your experimental design must show logical thinking

Your "Research Design and Methods" section is the most important part of your entire proposal, not only because it presents your specific goals, ideas, and experiments, but also because it showcases the way you think as a scientist. In addition to details, this section must convey an overall sense of logic, demonstrating to the reviewers that you have a clear line of reasoning and well thought-out plan.

You probably won't have room to create a summary diagram for every specific aim in your proposal, but your reviewers must be able to perceive the potential outcomes and associated conclusions for each experiment that you perform. You must also describe back-up plans in the case that your initial experiments don't work.

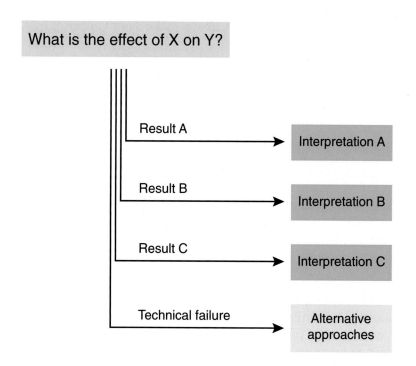

If your reviewers cannot perceive your logical thought process, your proposal will make less of an impact and will not be funded.

Enhance the visual design of your proposals

When you write a research or review article, your manuscript is typically 20–40 pages in length and, if accepted, will be reformatted by a page layout specialist prior to publication. In contrast, a research proposal is typically 5–10 pages in length and your target audience will see exactly what you submit to them with no improvements to the visual design.

The visual layout and design of your research proposal is highly important because it enhances the communication of your ideas, increases the perception of structure and logic, and implies clear, organized thinking.

Also consider that the typical reviewer critically examines four to eight research proposals during a single funding cycle. Reading dozens of pages of text eventually becomes tedious, and anything you can do to make your proposal more pleasing to read will be much appreciated.

Highlight your structure. Write all of your major headings (e.g., "Background and Significance," "Preliminary Data," "Research Design and Methods") in a larger font size, in bold, and in all capital letters. Also write all of your subheadings in bold.

Highlight your research hypothesis/goal. Both in your Executive Summary and at the end of your Background and Significance sections, write a clear, discrete sentence declaring your overall hypothesis or goal. Emphasize this sentence by underlining it or writing it in bold and/or italics.

Include as many diagrams as possible. Diagrams are visually interesting and communicate information very quickly. In research proposals, you might think of including explanatory diagrams to communicate your hypothesis/goal or any uncommon methods. Also consider using timelines or other useful diagrams to depict your experimental design.

Deliberately include empty space. Reviewers are turned off by too much text, especially if you use a relatively small font size and minimal margins. Separate your sections (or even individual paragraphs) with spacing and reduce wordiness as much as possible so you can increase the size of your margins and make your proposal more readable.

Before: tedious layout

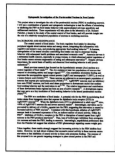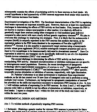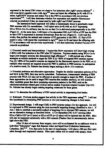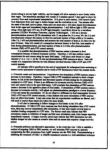

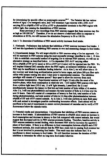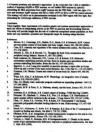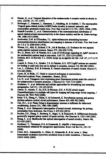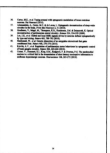

After: optimized layout to enhance communication

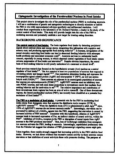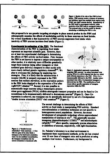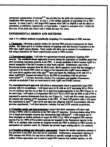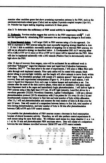

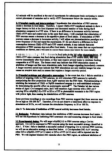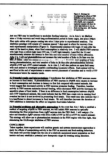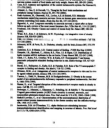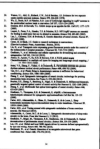

Summary: Design principles for writing research proposals

- The key task in writing a research proposal is to justify everything you state: justify why your scientific question is important, why you are the best person to perform the experiments, why you will succeed, why the results will be important, etc.

- When writing your research proposal, keep in mind the specific criteria used to evaluate proposals by the funding agency to which you submit. Write and edit each section of the proposal to try to attain the maximum score for each criterion.

- Ensure that your proposal is written such that the Background and Significance section directly leads into your specific hypothesis or goal. The background is really a long rationale as to why your proposed experiments are crucial and timely.

- Write your Research Design and Methods to highlight the rationale, experimental design, potential results and interpretations, and potential problems and alternative approaches for each of your specific aims.

- Ensure that the logic of your experimental design is completely obvious to the reviewers—that you have carefully thought out each potential experimental outcome and what conclusions you will make.

- To help your reviewers and improve visual communication, deliberately enhance the visual design of your proposals with bolded subheadings, a visibly distinctive hypothesis/goal, and as many diagrams as possible.

Part 4

Designing slide presentations

13

The use of slides in oral presentations

Slide presentations have become the most common way for scientists to share their ideas and work with others. Graduate students and postdocs typically publish 1–3 research articles and present 1–5 posters during each stage of their training. In contrast, they deliver dozens of slide presentations. The frequency of talks only increases at the faculty level, in which principal investigators present research seminars on the lecture circuit, speak at scientific meetings, and teach courses. With the use of slides so widespread, it is surprising that there is a general lack of training about their use in oral presentations. When used poorly, slides can mar a presentation, sabotage a speaker's message, and confuse an audience. However, when well-designed, slides add tremendous impact to a talk, enriching the information an audience receives and enhancing the visual communication of scientific ideas.

Designing Science Presentations. https://doi.org/10.1016/B978-0-12-815377-2.00013-5

The purpose of slides as presentation tools

Slides are so ubiquitous in oral presentations that most people don't even consider the possibility of delivering a talk without them. Whether we realize it or not, using slides in our presentations is a deliberate choice, and we often have the freedom to present talks with oral delivery alone. Therefore, it is worthwhile to ask, why do we use slides in oral presentations at all? What benefit do they provide our audiences?

As discussed often throughout this book, data are best conveyed visually in graphs and tables. Audiences don't just want to hear about the results and conclusions of experiments, they want to visualize data so that they can draw their own conclusions. Additionally, diagrams and photographs provide tremendous explanatory power. Therefore, visual aids are invaluable to good science presentations.

So why not use a handout instead of slides?

The power of slides as presentation tools is that they allow you to show your audience *whatever* you want them to see, *whenever* you want them to see it. Unlike a paper, poster, or handout, it is *you* who controls the flow of visual information in a presentation.

Without care and deliberation, the misuse of the power to control the flow of visual information can lead to confusing, unintelligible, and even annoying presentations. However, by making deliberate design decisions to help your audience, slides can offer much greater impact than your words alone.

Slides are for the audience, not the speaker

Perhaps the most common and unintentional mistake that people make when creating slide presentations is to compose slides for *themselves* rather than their audience. For example, they use slides as presentation notes so they know what to say during a talk and when to say it. They put visual elements on a slide that will remind them to explain a concept instead of to help audience members understand a concept. They allow templates and default settings to structure a talk for them without regard to the best narrative for their listeners.

Slides are best used to convey information, ideas, and emotions to an audience, not to save a presenter time and effort in delivering a presentation. If a presenter feels they can't present without slides, they are probably using them for the wrong reason.

The proof of the dependency of some presenters on their slides occurs when a computer crashes or a projector fails and the speaker suddenly has to deliver a presentation without slides. Everyone in the audience feels bad for the speaker instead of the other way around. If the speaker is a master of the content and has thoroughly thought through the needs of the audience, then they should be able to get through the presentation without slides. In fact, it should be the *presenter* who feels bad for the *audience* that they are denied a communication aid.

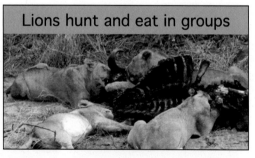

The slide on the left helps the speaker more than it helps the audience. All of this information can easily be conveyed orally without needing to be placed on a slide. In contrast, consider the immediate impact of the slide on the right. With this slide, the speaker can deliver the same information much more effectively.

Design a slide presentation from an audience's perspective

We may not consider ourselves experts at designing slide presentations, but we are all expert audience members. After the hundreds, if not thousands of slide presentations we have seen, we have many opinions about what we like and dislike in a talk.

The best overall strategy for designing an effective presentation is to consistently consider an audience's point of view, providing the kinds of experiences you would want if attending your own talk.

What audiences want from presentation design

- A rationale for why the topic is interesting and important
- An introduction that clearly explains what is necessary to know to understand the rest of the presentation
- Information presented one piece at a time
- Visual information that is clear and legible
- A balance of specific information with the overall big picture
- A chance to catch up if they momentarily lose attention
- A summary of what to remember after the talk is over

What audiences want from presentation delivery

- Interest and passion from the speaker
- A sense of expertise in the speaker
- A friendly, accessible speaker
- A speaker that can emphathize with the general mood of the audience
- A smooth technical delivery and use of technology
- A sense of how much a talk has progressed (and how much remains)
- A presentation that runs on time

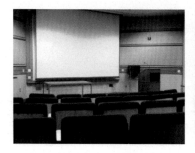 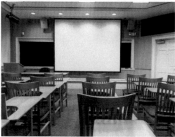

Have you ever tried designing a slide presentation in an empty lecture room? Literally sitting where your audience will sit can help you design a science presentation from an audience's perspective.

To design for your audience, know your audience

One of the most important factors that affects the success of a talk is a speaker's ability to connect with and understand their audience. Sometimes an otherwise excellent presentation fails because it doesn't conform to a particular group of people. Therefore, one of the first steps in designing a presentation should be to clearly define your target audience. Your scientific content may be exactly the same from presentation to presentation, but the format and delivery you choose can change from one audience to another. Presenting a science presentation to senior undergraduates in a packed lecture hall at 9:00 a.m. will require a different style and delivery than an invited seminar talk at a symposium attended by other scientists in your field at 4:00 p.m.

Different audiences have different needs, expectations, and attitudes, and designing a great presentation means designing a presentation with your specific audience in mind.

Questions to ask about your audience

Who are they?
What level of experience do they have for your subject matter? What is their average age or level of education? What are their interests? What are they likely to find exciting and what is likely to bore them?

Why are they attending your talk?
Is their attendance required or voluntary? What will they be looking for in your presentation? What do they hope to receive?

What do they need to know?
What background information is essential to present because they won't understand your talk without it?

What do they already know?
What background information is not necessary to present in detail because they are already likely to know it?

Do they hold any preconceptions or biases?
What opinions about your topic or field are they likely to have prior to the start of your talk? Why might they already object to information in your background or results?

What is their likely mood during your talk?
What time of day is your talk? Is your audience likely to be tired? Hungry? Anxious? Are they waiting for your talk to end so that they can go do something else?

Compose ideas before you compose slides

When using slide-making applications, there is a natural tendency to focus on slides rather than on ideas. After all, when you first open these applications, you see windows that look like this:

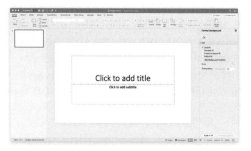

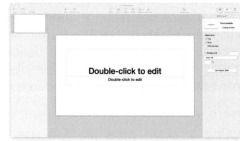

Microsoft PowerPoint user interface   Apple Keynote user interface

Big, blank slides with long, empty slide columns almost seem to beg you to fill them up with stuff. It is easy to find yourself going from blank slide to blank slide, filling them up one at a time until eventually all of your content is represented within the slide show. And it feels like such an accomplishment to have a complete slide deck that sometimes making slides becomes the goal in itself.

The problem with using blank slides as a starting point is that it changes the process by which you design a presentation. Rather than focusing on your content and the best ways to share ideas with an audience, you focus on slides as individual units, segmenting your information into bite-sized bits that may not be ideal for communication.

Before you even open a slide-making application, outline the structure of your presentation and organize the order and importance of your ideas. Concepts that you especially want to emphasize may take more than one slide to communicate.

Instead of designing slides in a way that is slide-centric, design in a way that is idea-centric.

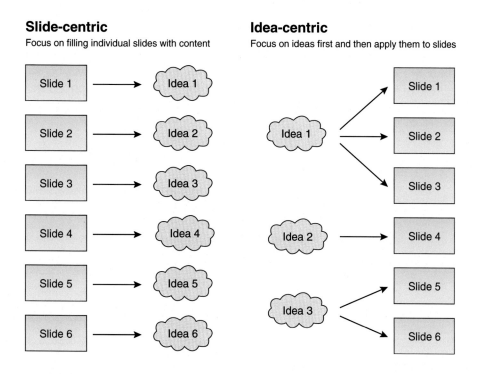

Slide-centric
Focus on filling individual slides with content

Idea-centric
Focus on ideas first and then apply them to slides

Research into the use of slides as presentation tools has demonstrated that presentations made in a slide-centric way can actually obscure information. In his 32-page essay, *The Cognitive Style of PowerPoint: Pitching Out Corrupts Within*, Edward Tufte, a pioneer in the field of data visualization, suggests that slide-making applications themselves can change the way that people conceive of and deliver information. The solution is to focus on ideas and content, rather than the slides themselves.

The relationship between slides and oral delivery

During a slide presentation, audiences receive information from two different sources: your voice, and your slides. When your narration and visuals complement each other, you achieve a great harmony that helps your audience understand your content. When narration and visuals contrast, your audience can become distracted and confused.

Your oral narration is what drives your presentation forward, and visual aids are always subservient to what you say. Choose visual content that emphasizes and clarifies what you say out loud, not the other way around.

Everything that you say doesn't need to be on a slide. Only show something on a slide if it will help your audience to understand or better appreciate what you say in your delivery. In contrast, anything presented on a slide should be presented in your oral delivery. Therefore, if there is something on a slide that you aren't actually going to talk about, get rid of it.

Before

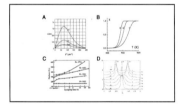

After

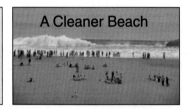

Not all information needs to be communicated visually. Cutting text that you can easily convey orally allows you to emphasize visual information that is most important.

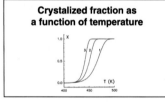

In contrast, anything you are displaying on a slide should be explained in your oral delivery. Therefore, if you're only talking about a single part of a detailed figure, get rid of all the parts you aren't actively explaining.

There is no correct number of slides

There is a common myth that you should compose about one slide for every minute of a presentation. In reality, there is no formula that calculates the time your talk will take to deliver based on the number of slides in your presentation. How long you typically spend delivering slides depends on your delivery style and your content. Some excellent presenters use only 20 slides over the course of an hour-long talk and the audience is never bored. Others use hundreds of slides and the audience never feels rushed. It all depends on you and your content.

There is no golden rule about how many slides to use in a presentation except to know yourself and your own speaking style. The only way to truly know the length of your presentation is to rehearse.

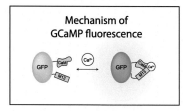 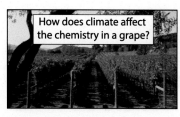 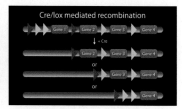

Depending on how the speaker presents the subject matter of these slides, each may take several minutes to explain and discuss.

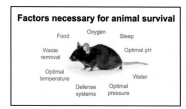 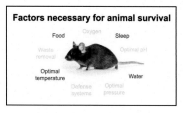 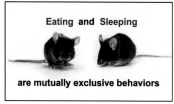

These three slides, when presented in succession and accompanied with a good oral delivery, might make a point in less than minute.

Exceptional slide presentations require time and effort

Making a mediocre slide presentation is really easy … all you have to do is wait until the day before a presentation, open a slide-making application, create a bunch of slides, and deliver them with some memory of their order. If you're lucky, you won't have any obvious typos. However, designing an effective slide presentation is hard work. Consider the amount of time you might spend:

Time estimates for designing an effective slide presentation

Analyze data: 5-50 hours
Sort data in spreadsheets, perform quantitative and statistical analyses, etc.

Design elegant graphs, tables, diagrams, and photos: 5-20 hours
Produce data graphics and infographics and optimize all visual elements for a slide presentation.

Research relevant background information: 1-10 hours
Peruse the scientific literature to find key background papers, figures, etc. for your audience.

Brainstorm and outline the narrative of the presentation: 1-8 hours
Organize your information into a scientific story and simultaneously translate your content into an oral delivery and slide presentation.

Design slides: 5-50 hours
Use a slide-making application to translate your ideas into a visual story.

Edit slides: 1-5 hours
Proceed through your presentation, one slide at a time, optimizing visual elements, layout, and animations.

Rehearse: 1-3 hours
Practice your delivery in whatever way works best for you: in front of a practice audience, by yourself, on your bike, in the shower, etc.

Test your slide show in a presentation room with a projector: 1-2 hours
Calibrate a laptop with projector settings and ensure that projected slides appear correctly.

Total time: 20-150 hours

These time estimates assume you are creating a presentation completely from scratch. In reality, you may recycle much of one presentation for another, and some presentations are much shorter than others. The amount of time you should dedicate to designing a presentation is proportional to the importance of the talk, however, all presentations require time and effort. Designing a presentation for a professional meeting, invited seminar, job talk, thesis defense, etc., will require many hours, perhaps several days of work. Even presentations that are less consequential (e.g., lab meetings, journal clubs) are important because they establish your reputation among your peers and colleagues.

Summary: Design principles for using slides

- Slides are powerful presentation tools because they allow you to show your audience whatever you want them to see, whenever you want them to see it. Unlike other presentation formats, you are in total control of the flow of visual information.

- Many presenters unconsciously create slides to help them remember what to say during a talk. Always remember that slides are for the audience, not the speaker.

- Design presentations with your audience in mind. Think about their backgrounds, needs, experiences, attitudes, and even their likely state of mind during your presentation. Provide the kinds of experiences you would want if you were attending your own talk.

- Compose ideas before you compose slides. Don't make the mistake of filling slide after slide with content before you have had a chance to outline your content first. Design slides in a way that is idea-centric and not slide-centric.

- It is always okay to orally convey information without representing it on a slide. Some information is naturally best presented visually or emphasized with your speech and slides, but much information can probably be best conveyed with your narration alone.

- In contrast, everything visually displayed on a slide should be discussed. To reduce distractions, omit all visual items from a slide that you aren't going to talk about.

- There is no magic number of slides that one should include for a talk of a specific length. Some slides can be presented in seconds, others will take several minutes to fully explain. The only way to know the length of your slide presentation is to rehearse.

- Exceptional slide presentations require much time and effort to prepare. When designing a presentation from scratch, a slide presentation might take anywhere from 20 to 150 h, depending on if you have already analyzed data, made figures, or created slides for other talks.

14

The structure of a slide presentation

When designing a slide presentation from scratch, many people tend to focus on what their slides will look like. Just as important, if not more so, is the structure of a presentation—the organization of ideas and concepts into a larger scientific story. Telling a story with a beginning, middle, and end, especially including a good rationale for a scientific project and how it fits into a larger body of knowledge, helps audiences appreciate not just facts and data but a larger sense of context. Scientists who tell stories create better experiences for their audiences, increasing attention, comprehension, and overall impact.

Designing Science Presentations. https://doi.org/10.1016/B978-0-12-815377-2.00014-7

A good scientific talk is a good scientific story

Science presentations have a surprising amount in common with action movies. Although great action scenes, special effects, and outrageous stunts are fun to watch, nobody wants to see a movie composed entirely of action with no character or plot development. In fact, movies composed entirely of action and explosions with no story can actually bore audiences.

Similarly, a common problem with many science presentations is a narrow focus on experiments and data. While data and results are obviously the core of any science talk, audiences often lose interest if experiments aren't framed as part of a larger scientific story.

Audiences don't just want to see data, they want to hear a complete scientific story with a beginning, middle, and end. The beginning conveys a rationale, sense of importance, and a clear goal. The middle contains the experiments, results and conclusion. The end provides a sense of resolution, places your results in a larger scientific context, and looks to the future.

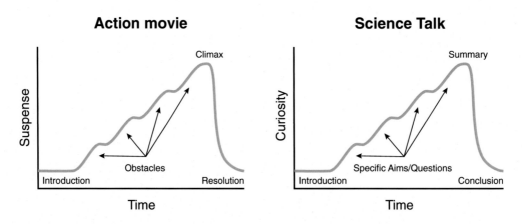

A typical plot diagram for an action movie can be similar to a the narrative structure of a scientific presentation. Just as a protagonist overcomes obstacles through a series of action scenes, a scientist pursues scientific objectives through a series of experiments to reach a goal. As a scientist comes closer and closer to reaching a goal, curiosity comes to a maximal point, the initial scientific question is answered, and the presentation reaches a sense of resolution.

Good science stories should convey the scientific method

Most people learn the scientific method early in their education, perhaps in elementary school or middle school. While it is relatively easy to appreciate the scientific method as a kid, it is also easy to become distracted by the exciting, dazzling complexity of our scientific fields as we pursue training in college, graduate school, and beyond. When talking about science, sometimes we can be susceptible of focusing on the exciting concepts and methodology of our fields while forgetting to convey the scientific process. Sometimes we are so excited to share our results that we forget to place those results in the context of the scientific method.

A good science presentation always presents information in the context of the scientific method, even if the scientific method is not explicitly referred to during a talk. There should always be a sense of the background knowledge, hypothesis/goal, methods, and discussion to frame results in a larger scientific context.

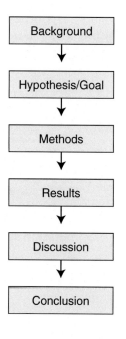

No matter your specific scientific field, no matter how exciting your methods or results, a good science presentation should contain all elements of the scientific method.

Even if you are presenting to highly experienced scientists in your field, try to channel what you learned about the scientific process as a kid. Providing the context behind your work will only enhance the complex information you share.

Consider storyboarding a talk to preview its structure

Storyboarding is a technique used by filmmakers and animators to quickly preview how a media project will look and feel prior to spending time and money actually executing the project. Sometimes it is immediately obvious that an idea that sounds good on paper doesn't come off as intended in its final form. Additionally, storyboarding allows an artist to realize problems in advance and make decisions that will affect and unify an entire production.

Like a filmmaker, a scientist can quickly storyboard a talk to preview the pacing, storytelling, color schemes, and delivery. No artistic skills are required, and the beauty of storyboarding is that you can outline several slides in minutes.

An effective way to storyboard is to first list all of the content you want to cover in a presentation, then to produce a very rough sketch of what those slides will look like in final form.

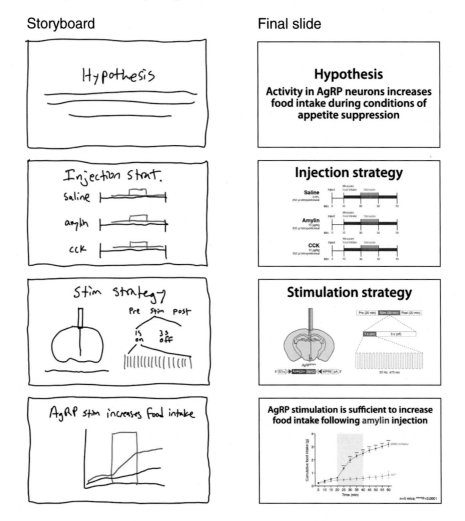

Set the tone of your talk with a title slide

Your scientific story begins before you even begin speaking.

Title slides are more than just token beginnings to slide presentations. Consider that your title slide will probably be the slide that your audience looks at for the longest amount of time, from the moment they sit down to the moment you are introduced. Therefore, you can use these slides to communicate information without costing you time during your actual talk. Besides introducing details about yourself, you can use a title slide to set a tone for the rest of your presentation to follow.

A good title slide contains:

- **A good title.** Good presentation titles inform an audience of exactly what to expect from a talk.

- **Your name and affiliation.** Let people know who you are, even at internal retreats in which many people are likely to know you.

- **The date and function of the talk.** Writing the date and function will convey that you designed the talk specifically for *this* audience and *this* venue.

- **A picture or diagram that sets the tone.** Including a picture or diagram will psychologically prepare your audience for the subject matter of your talk before you even say a word.

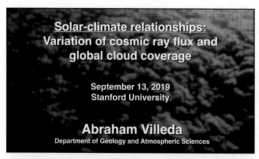

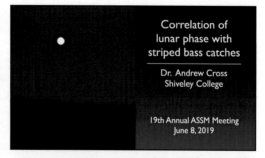

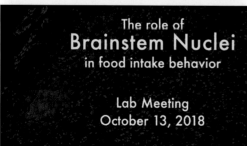

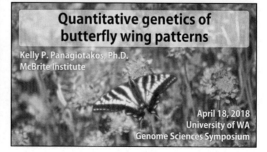

Start a talk by progressing from general questions to specific goals

It is jarring for an audience when a speaker begins with highly detailed, specific information. Even people who are familiar with your work or research topic will appreciate being gradually led from a broad question or problem to a specific scientific goal.

To attract the interest of everyone in your audience, always start a presentation with a statement or question that anyone from any discipline should be able to understand and appreciate. Gradually focus your introduction toward your specific topic and research goal, defining specific terminology and concepts that people might not understand.

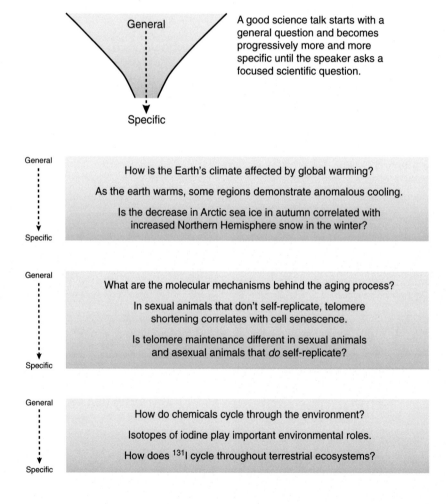

A good science talk starts with a general question and becomes progressively more and more specific until the speaker asks a focused scientific question.

General
⋮
Specific

How is the Earth's climate affected by global warming?

As the earth warms, some regions demonstrate anomalous cooling.

Is the decrease in Arctic sea ice in autumn correlated with increased Northern Hemisphere snow in the winter?

General
⋮
Specific

What are the molecular mechanisms behind the aging process?

In sexual animals that don't self-replicate, telomere shortening correlates with cell senescence.

Is telomere maintenance different in sexual animals and asexual animals that *do* self-replicate?

General
⋮
Specific

How do chemicals cycle through the environment?

Isotopes of iodine play important environmental roles.

How does ^{131}I cycle throughout terrestrial ecosystems?

Clearly emphasize your scientific goal and why it is worth pursuing

Before learning about any specific experiments or results, audiences want to know the answers to two questions: what is your ultimate scientific goal, and why is reaching that goal important?

When speakers do not clearly articulate a question or goal that drives their research, their data and results lack context: the audience may understand specific experiments, but not how the results fit into a bigger picture. When speakers do not explain a rationale for their experiments, their results don't seem interesting. The audience may understand what the speaker did, but not why they should care.

Before presenting any data, clearly state and emphasize your overarching scientific goal and why reaching that goal is interesting. If you don't state your goal in the beginning, your audience won't know if you reached it at the end. And if you don't state your rationale in the beginning, your audience won't *care* if you reached it at the end.

Before

> ## AgRP Neurons
>
> - Activity increases when animals are hungry
> - Respond to circulating satiety and hunger signals (glucose, leptin, insulin, ghrelin)
> - Antagonize aMSH on anorexigenic MC4R-bearing neurons
> - What is the effect of ablating AgRP neurons on food-seeking behavior?

After

> ### AgRP neurons play a major role in food-seeking behavior
>
> - They increase activity when animals are hungry
> - They respond to circulating satiety and hunger signals
> - They antagonize anorexigenic MC4R-bearing neurons

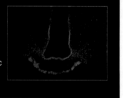

> ### What is the effect of ablating AgRP neurons on food-seeking behavior?

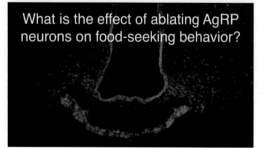

In the slide on the left, the major question that drives the entire research study is buried at the bottom of a text-heavy slide. Any audience member who is not paying full attention may miss that the central research question was even mentioned. A better way to emphasize the research question is to separate it from the background information and place it on its own slide. Adding an attractive photograph or diagram increases audience interest so that everyone clearly understands the research question throughout the rest of the talk.

Prepare for inevitable shifts in attention

Audiences rarely focus their complete attention on a science presentation throughout the entire talk. They may start out actively listening to what you say, but they inevitably become distracted and lose attention as your talk becomes more detailed. These distractions are natural—we are all human, and full concentration is difficult to maintain, especially for presentations that last an hour or more. Even the best presenters occasionally lose parts of their audience.

One of your design goals in structuring a scientific talk is to prepare for the inevitable periods during which your audience is likely to become distracted.

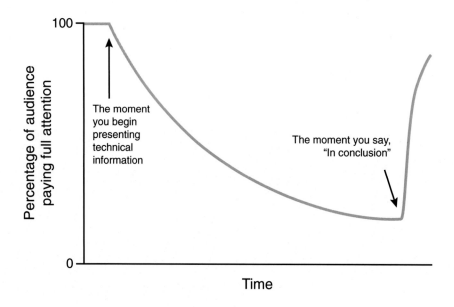

Predict the moments during which people are likely to break concentration and deliberately structure your presentation so that you employ methods, described on the following pages, of maintaining and regaining their attention.

Organize the presentation of data into individual segments

After delivering background information to their audiences, many scientists present detailed scientific information (experiments, methods, results) in one long continuous section until they reach the end of their talk. During these long stretches of technical detail, audiences often become unfocused and gradually stop paying attention. In presentations that last longer than 10–15 min, even the most interested scientists need mental breaks. Instead of presenting data all at once, organize your information into more manageable segments.

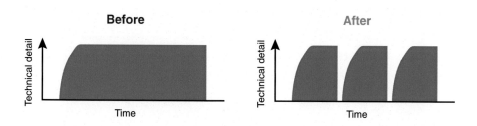

After each segment of data, give your audience a brief break—not a literal pause in your talk, but a pause in the presentation of detailed information. During this pause you can:

- Summarize what you just covered
- Ask if there are any questions
- Connect the details of your data with the larger scientific story
- Provide interesting examples/applications of what you just covered
- Tell a relevant anecdote or humorous story
- Show a video clip likely to recapture audience attention

By providing these pauses in data, you not only allow your audience to catch their breath after a stretch of detailed information, you also balance details with the big picture, integrating the results of experiments with your larger scientific story.

Consider uniting sections of a talk using a "home slide"

When dividing a longer presentation (a presentation over 10–15 min) into manageable segments, it can be helpful to your audience to provide an outline that follows the structure of your talk and tracts your progress throughout. This outline can be provided in the form of a *home slide*—a slide you return to throughout your talk to unite different segments into a cohesive whole.

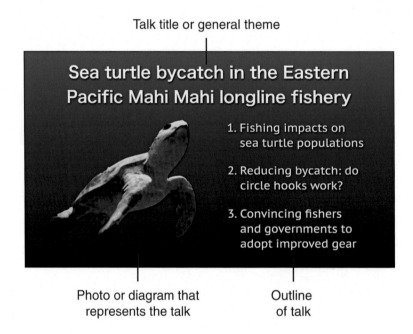

A good home slide contains an outline of the different sections of your talk with a picture or unifying diagram that represents the big picture. Show this slide before you present your first segment of data and at the end of every section until the conclusion of your talk. Using a home slide between sections helps your audience understand where they are in the course of your talk. You can also return to your home slide at the end of your presentation to summarize all of the information you covered.

How often should you refer to your home slide throughout your talk? For a 45-min talk, you might divide your data into two to four segments and use a home slide three to five times. While using this slide multiple times may seem repetitive to you, your audience will appreciate the obvious exposition of structure.

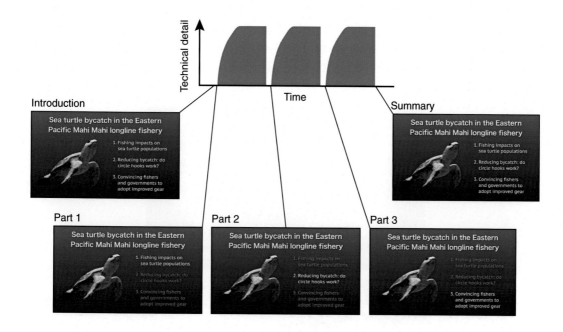

Deliberately emphasize one to three take-home messages

It can sometimes be depressing to realize that just hours after a presentation ends, most audience members will forget all but a few details of your talk. You can help your audience by directly telling them what details you especially hope they will remember. These details can be key findings from your results, or even an overall conclusion about your work.

If you want your audience to remember one or two key aspects of your talk, deliberately highly these items when they are most salient. Telling your audience what is important to you will make those items resonate long after your talk is over.

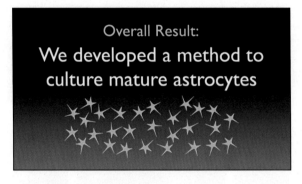

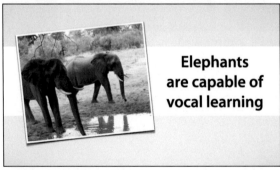

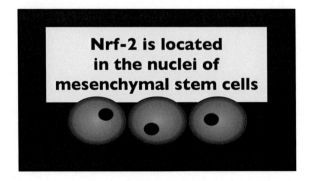

Conclude a talk by transitioning from specific details to a broader scientific context

Just as you begin a talk by transitioning from general ideas into your specific scientific results, end a presentation by transitioning from your experiments and results to broader conclusions. Ending on a general note will help your audience understand how your work fits into a larger scientific objective and how your findings could lead to bigger, broader outcomes.

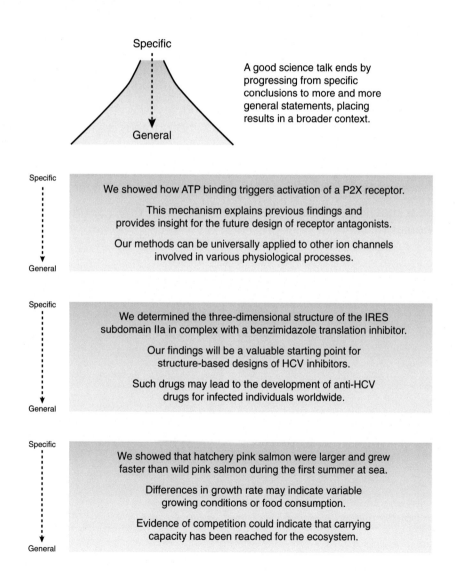

Specific

General

A good science talk ends by progressing from specific conclusions to more and more general statements, placing results in a broader context.

Specific

General

We showed how ATP binding triggers activation of a P2X receptor.

This mechanism explains previous findings and provides insight for the future design of receptor antagonists.

Our methods can be universally applied to other ion channels involved in various physiological processes.

Specific

General

We determined the three-dimensional structure of the IRES subdomain IIa in complex with a benzimidazole translation inhibitor.

Our findings will be a valuable starting point for structure-based designs of HCV inhibitors.

Such drugs may lead to the development of anti-HCV drugs for infected individuals worldwide.

Specific

General

We showed that hatchery pink salmon were larger and grew faster than wild pink salmon during the first summer at sea.

Differences in growth rate may indicate variable growing conditions or food consumption.

Evidence of competition could indicate that carrying capacity has been reached for the ecosystem.

Briefly acknowledge your contributors

Scientists often conclude their presentations with a slide that acknowledges the contributions of others and their funding sources. It is always important and considerate to acknowledge the people, organizations, and funders who helped make your science and presentation possible. However, just like the end credits at the end of a movie, acknowledgments typically don't have much value for an audience. In fact, when a speaker displays an acknowledgments slide, most audience members immediately stop paying attention. Definitely acknowledge your colleagues and funding sources—but try not to spend too long presenting long lists of names that many people probably won't even recognize. Succinctly acknowledge your contributors, then move on.

Tips for acknowledging your coworkers:

- Try not to spend more than 20–30 s on an acknowledgments slide.

- Display a photograph of your lab, the key individuals who contributed to your work, or the city/institution where you are located. Photographs are more exciting to look at than lists of names.

- Don't read through long lists of names that most people probably won't recognize. Highlight a few key individuals, but don't read the names of everyone in your lab.

- Instead of acknowledging everyone at the end of your talk, consider acknowledging key individuals throughout your presentation when appropriate. But only briefly!

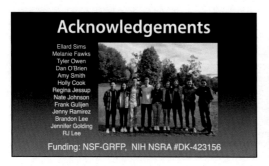 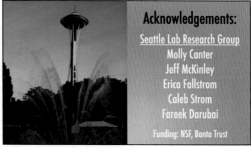

Answer questions while showing a summary diagram

Most scientific talks typically end with a brief question-and-answer period. During this time, presenters usually either exit their slide shows or continue to display their acknowledgments slides. Consider a third option: while answering questions, display a slide that contains a simple summary of your talk. This slide can be your home slide, or perhaps an optimized version that displays the overall conclusion of your experiments. Showing a summary diagram will help make your talk more memorable and even help your audience ask better questions because all of the relevant information will be in front of them.

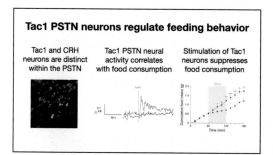

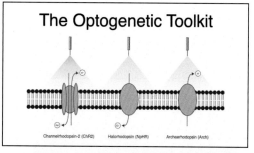

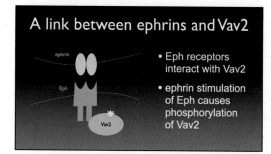

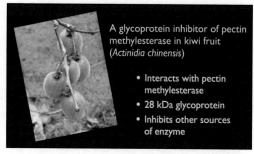

Example outline of a structured talk

Here is an abridged example of the structure you might use for a scientific talk. Each of the slides below might represent one or several slides that you create for an actual presentation. Don't let this outline make you think that a structured talk has to seem typical or routine … just like learning the steps in a dance routine, having structure actually promotes expression and creativity rather than providing a rigid set of rules.

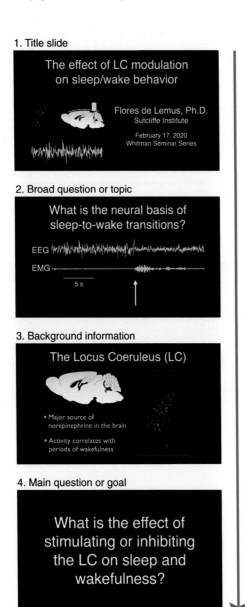

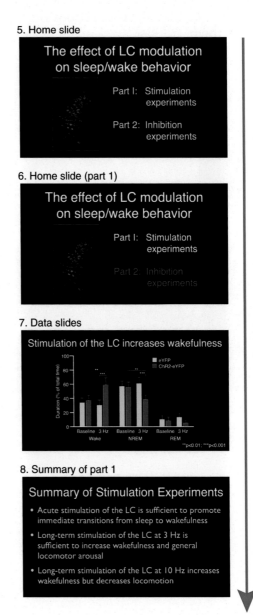

9. Home slide (part 2)

The effect of LC modulation on sleep/wake behavior

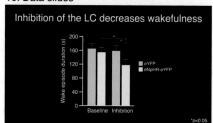

Part I: Stimulation
          experiments

Part 2: Inhibition
          experiments

10. Data slides

Inhibition of the LC decreases wakefulness

eYFP
eNpHR-eYFP

Wake episode duration (s)

200
160
120
80
40
0

Baseline   Inhibition

*p<0.05

11. Summary of part 2

Summary of Inhibition Experiments

- The LC is necessary for normal maintenance of wakefulness states during the active period
- Inhibition of the LC increases slow-wave activity in the EEG towards the end of wake bouts
- The LC is necessary for Hcrt-mediated sleep-to-wake transitions

12. Home slide

The effect of LC modulation on sleep/wake behavior

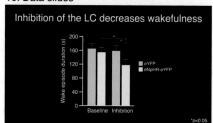

Part I: Stimulation
          experiments

Part 2: Inhibition
          experiments

13. Conclusion

Conclusion: The LC is necessary for normal durations of wakefulness and sufficient to promote wakefulness

14. Broad ending

Potential role of LC in network with other subcortical nuclei

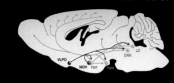

VLPO
MCH Hcrt
TMN
LC
DRN

15. Acknowledgements

Acknowledgments

The de Lemus lab:
  Mark Duncan
  Evan Matthews ——
  Lindsey O'Brien
  Yakima Grey
  Pacey Carter
  Anne Bloit

Needs a jolt to the LC!

16. Question and answer

The effect of LC modulation on sleep/wake behavior

Stimulation of the LC increases wakefulness

Inhibition of the LC decreases wakefulness

Summary: Design principles for slide presentation structure

- When designing a slide presentation, start by thinking about your presentation's structure before thinking about the visual design of the slides themselves.

- Audiences don't want to see a presentation composed only of experiments and data. Every presentation should tell a story and place scientific results in a larger context.

- A good presentation conveys the scientific method, even if the scientific method is not explicitly referenced.

- Consider storyboarding a talk to preview the pacing, storytelling, color schemes, and delivery. No artistic skills are necessary, and storyboarding a talk can be completed in minutes.

- To help your audience become excited for your talk before it starts, start your presentation with a title slide that contains your title, name and affiliation, date and function of your talk, and a picture or diagram that sets the tone.

- Start a talk by talking about general concepts that anyone can understand and appreciate, and then gradually transition into your focused topic and goal.

- Clearly emphasize your scientific goal and why it is worth pursuing. If you don't state your goal in the beginning, your audience won't know if you reached it in the end. And if you don't state a rationale, your audience won't care if you reached it at the end.

- Prepare for the fact that it is natural for audience members to lose attention the longer a talk goes on. Deliberately use strategies to regain audience attention at key moments during your talk.

- To help your audience pay attention and balance details with the big picture, organize your data into individual segments with breaks in between. Use these pauses to summarize what you just covered and connect details with a larger scientific story.

- For longer presentations, consider uniting various aspects of a talk with a home slide, a slide you return to throughout your talk to unite different segments into a cohesive whole.

- Conclude a talk by transitioning from specific details to a broader scientific context that shows how your project fits into bigger, broader outcomes.

- To help your audience remember your talk and ask better questions, show a summary diagram of your project during the question and answer period.

15

Visual elements in slide presentations

Compared to a written document or scientific poster, the useable surface area of a presentation slide is relatively small. In a single slide, you only have room to display a handful of visual elements: a title, one or two figures, and some minimal text. Because the number of visual elements that can and should be used per slide is low, the design choices you make about each are highly consequential for the overall clarity and impact of your presentation.

Designing Science Presentations. https://doi.org/10.1016/B978-0-12-815377-2.00015-9

Optimizing visual elements on slides

Individual presentation slides have the lowest resolution of any presentation format. To avoid overwhelming a single slide with too much content, there is only room for some minimal text and a very small number of other visual elements.

A typical slide only contains a few of the following ingredients:

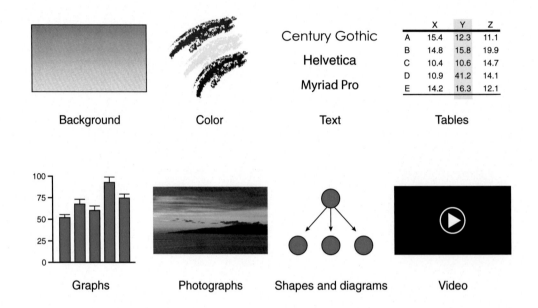

Background   Color   Text   Tables

Graphs   Photographs   Shapes and diagrams   Video

Because there are only a modest number of elements that constitute a slide, the design choices you make about each can greatly affect the clarity of your information and tone of your presentation.

Optimizing visual elements for slides is like choosing the best ingredients for a simple recipe: because you only use a few items, the quality of those ingredients has a tremendous impact on the final product. Likewise, the more you use design principles to optimize visual elements, the better you communicate information to an audience.

Add design instead of decoration

When creating a presentation from scratch, the sight of a blank, empty slide can sometimes cause us to fall into the trap of decorating rather than designing. We have a natural tendency to want to fill the slide with *stuff*, adding visual elements so that the slide doesn't appear empty. Additionally, when we see a slide that seems too simple, we have an urge to add color, ornamentation, and special effects.

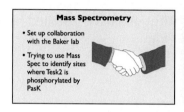 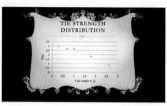 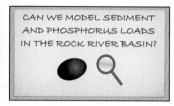

The problem with this way of thinking is that it ignores the entire purpose of creating a slide in the first place: to help present information to an audience.

Instead of adding decoration to a slide, add design. Decoration may help fill a slide, but designing a slide to communicate with your audience adds meaning and value.

Before

After

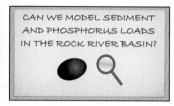

Choose the most optimal slide size for your screen/projector

When digital slides replaced photographic slides as the dominant form of slide presentation tool, all slides existed in a 4:3 aspect ratio. Correspondingly, projectors and screens were installed and optimized in presentation rooms and lecture halls for 4:3 slides.

Because desktop and laptop screens have became larger over the years, nowadays all feature a widescreen, high definition format. In turn, presentation applications have also offered the option for a widescreen 16:9 size. In fact, in most slide-making applications, 16:9 is now the default size. Therefore, many institutions have installed high definition projectors and installed wider screens for 16:9 slides.

4:3 standard slide

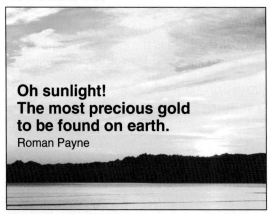

16:9 widescreen slide

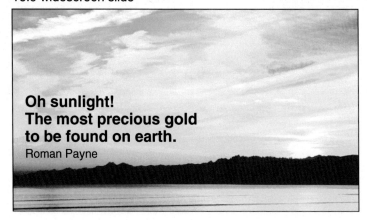

The decision of whether to present 4:3 or 16:9 slides is entirely based on the projector and screen size of the presentation room. If a 4:3 slide is presented in a room optimized for 16:9 slides, the slide will appear the same size, however, the presenter loses the opportunity for extra room on each side. If a 16:9 slide is presented in a room optimized for 4:3 slides, the slide will need to shrink to fit the screen, and the presenter will lose the opportunity for extra room on the top and bottom of each slide.

Therefore, when designing slides for a specific presentation, find out whether the room you will be speaking in is optimized for standard or widescreen slides. Many conferences now post presentation guidelines for creating slides, and if you are invited to give a talk at another institution, you can ask your host whether the presentation room is optimized for 4:3 or 16:9 slides.

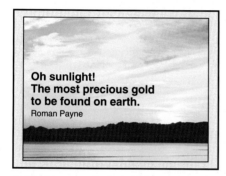

A 4:3 slide presented on a 4:3 screen.

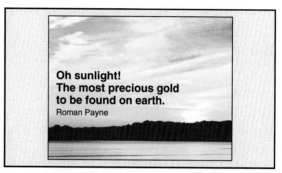

A 4:3 slide presented on a 16:9 widescreen will appear just as large, but the presenter loses the opportunity to expand the visual area on each side.

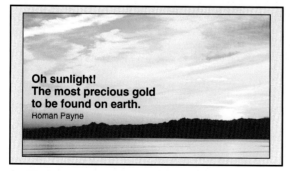

A 16:9 slide presented on a 16:9 widescreen.

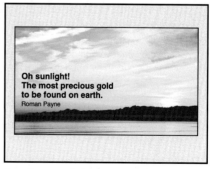

A projector optimized for a 4:3 screen will shrink a 16:9 slide to fit the screen. Therefore, the presenter effectively loses space on the top and bottom of the screen, and various aspects of the slide, such as the text, become smaller.

Choose inconspicuous backgrounds

The best slide backgrounds are just that: backgrounds that, by themselves, lack visual content.

Before

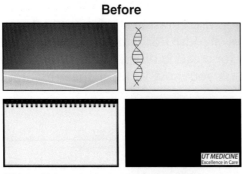

After

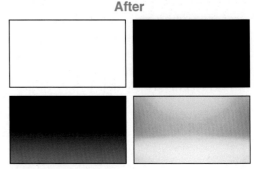

Slides with busy backgrounds reduce the amount of space you have for your own visual elements.

Slides with clear backgrounds allow you to fill the entire space with your own content.

Before

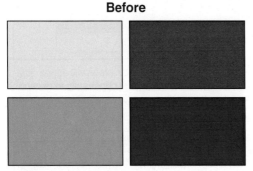

After

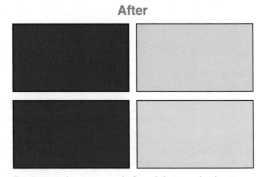

Backgrounds composed of warm, bright colors can be too intense on the eye and don't allow foreground objects to stand out.

Backgrounds composed of cool tints or shades are comfortable to look at for long time periods.

When choosing a background, consider how your charts and photographs will appear when placed in the foreground.

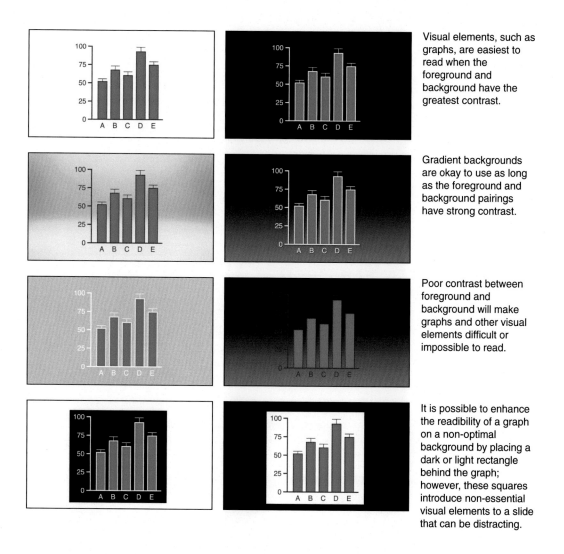

Visual elements, such as graphs, are easiest to read when the foreground and background have the greatest contrast.

Gradient backgrounds are okay to use as long as the foreground and background pairings have strong contrast.

Poor contrast between foreground and background will make graphs and other visual elements difficult or impossible to read.

It is possible to enhance the readibility of a graph on a non-optimal background by placing a dark or light rectangle behind the graph; however, these squares introduce non-essential visual elements to a slide that can be distracting.

Whatever background you choose, be consistent throughout your presentation. Jumping back and forth between different backgrounds is distracting and can be hard on the eyes.

Optimize color choices for slides

As discussed in Chapter 3, color should always be used deliberately and judiciously, either to emphasize a message or to set a tone.

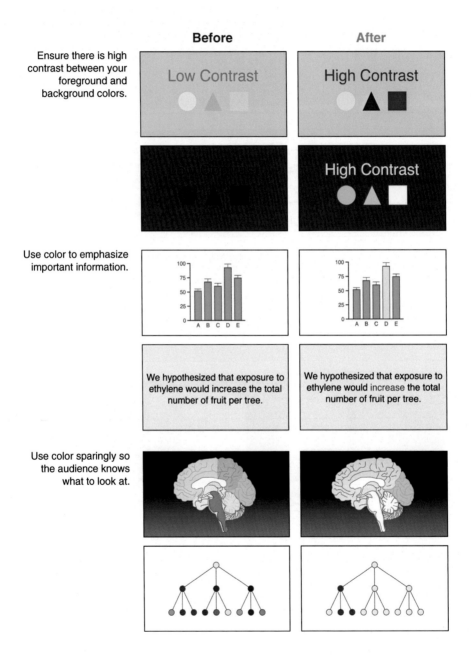

Assemble a unifying tone using a color palette

Depending on the occasion of your talk, you often have the freedom to use a greater combination of colors than you would for a more formal written or poster presentation. Different color schemes (called "color palettes") can set a unifying tone for your presentation while affecting the atmosphere and mood of your talk. There are hundreds of color palettes embedded in many photograph or illustrator applications (e.g., Photoshop and Illustrator), and you can find thousands online. To find great color palettes on the internet, simply search for "color palette" and some terms that are applicable to your presentation topic.

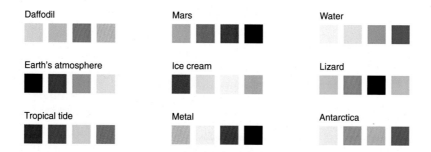

You can also design your own color palettes using your own photographs or photographs you find online. When choosing colors for your palette, identify a range of colors from light to dark so that you can create optimal foreground/background combinations. Whichever colors you choose, make sure that you are consistent across your presentation to unify the tone of your talk.

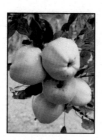

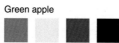

Green apple

The photograph on the left was used to produce this custom-made color palette. In this example, the lightest color was used as the background and the darkest colors were used for foreground elements. This color scheme is used consistently throughout the entire presentation.

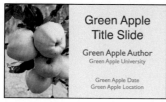

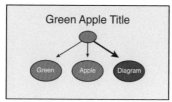

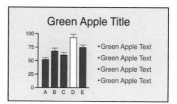

Choose fonts that are most legible

As discussed in Chapter 4, the most important consideration when making decisions about fonts and typography is optimizing legibility, especially legibility across a presentation room.

	Before	After

Any text you write on a slide should be legible in the back of the room. Even smaller text such as citations or footnotes should be legible in the back row.

Can you read this in the back of the room?

Carter (2020)

Can you read this in the back of the room?

Carter (2020)

Serif fonts are harder to read from a distance than sans serif fonts.

Serif fonts are more difficult to read from a distance

Overly complex fonts are nearly impossible to read from a distance

Sans serif fonts are easy to read from a distance

Helvetica

Myriad Pro

Century Gothic

Tahoma

To emphasize specific text within a slide, write the text in bold, italics, or a different color instead of underlining or writing in all caps.

On a slide, it is more difficult to read underlined words or words in ALL CAPS

If you want to emphasize a word, use **bold letters**, *italics*, or a different color

Keep text to a minimum

Probably the most common design problem in most slide presentations is too much text on one slide. If you find yourself filling up an entire slide with text, you really aren't designing slides for an audience, you are writing a document. Audiences don't enjoy reading long stretches of text … they are much more engaged by visual elements such as graphs, diagrams, and photos.

Try your best to keep text to a minimum. Adding more and more words to a slide increases the likelihood that your audience will stop paying attention.

A common mistake…

- How many times have you seen a slide like this? Probably too often.
- The use of too much text on one slide is so common that many of us don't even think to question it.
- If presenters are going to write out everything they are going to say during their delivery, then what is the point of attending their presentations? They might as well send their slides to us over email and we can read them whenever we want.

…but no less annoying.

- Seriously, slides like this are awful. Especially when every slide in the entire presentation looks like this.
- Too much text on a slide is one of the top reasons why audiences stop paying attention.
- One hundred years ago, movie studios realized that silent movies shouldn't contain too much dialogue because audiences didn't enjoy reading text on a screen. You'd think we would have learned the same concept in slide presentations by now.…

Even for complex scientific talks, when it comes to text…

The simpler, the better!

Less is more!

Minimize the use of lists and outlines

Scientists have many reasons to use lists in presentations: to present a set of facts, to describe the results of multiple published studies, to write steps in a process or procedure, to show all the outcomes of an experiment, etc. Outlines are a special category of lists with headings and subheadings (and sometimes sub-subheadings) that organize and sort information into logical groups.

The problem with including lists and outlines on slides is that they are tedious to look at, and audiences quickly lose attention when presented with long stretches of text.

Lists aren't very fun to look at

Monotonous	Lackluster
Tedious	Mundane
Dull	Tiresome
Boring	Irksome
Flat	Featureless
Bland	Colorless
Dry	Lifeless
Stale	Unvaried
Jejune	Humdrum
Vapid	Unexciting
Banal	Insipid

Neither are outlines

- This is the first major heading of an outline
  - Here is a subheading
  - Here is another subheading
- This is the second major heading of an outline
  - Here is a subheading
  - Here is another subheading
    - Sub-subheadings!
    - Sub-subheadings!
- This is the third major heading of an outline
  - Here is a subheading
  - Here is another subheading

To increase audience attention and engagement, try your best to minimize the use of lists in slide presentations, and try not to use outlines altogether. Instead of listing multiple facts or background studies on the same slide, consider breaking them up into several slides. Instead of presenting multiple items in one long list, consider splitting them up into different categories that are more manageable for an audience to comprehend.

FOXO Target Genes

AgRP	GADD45
Bim-1	MnSOD
Catalase	NPY
DDB1	p27
FasL	p130
G6Pase	PEPCK

FOXO Target Genes

ROS detoxification	DNA repair	Glucose metabolism
Catalase	GADD45	G6Pase
MnSOD	DDB1	PEPCK

Cell cycle arrest	Cell Death	Energy homeostasis
p27	Bim-1	AgRP
p130	FasL	NPY
GADD45		

Use slide titles to make a point

Most people place titles on the top of their slides because slide-making applications suggest making titles in their default settings. From a designer's point of view, make sure that every title has a deliberate purpose. Instead of making a title, make a point. Emphasize the message contained in your slide with brief text that conveys an unmistakable conclusion.

Before   **After**

Use a title to make a point, such as when presenting results, background information, ideas, etc.

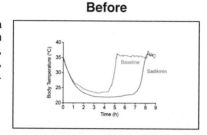 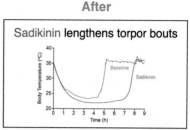

Don't use generic words or phrases like "Results," "Background," or "Conclusion." Instead, try to be specific about the larger point you want to emphasize.

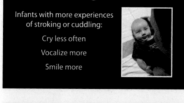 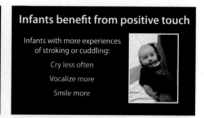

Don't feel that you need to use a slide title when the contents of a slide are obvious from a photograph or your oral narration.

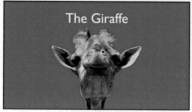 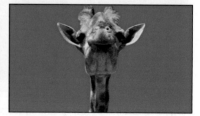

Optimize tables and graphs for slides

Scientists often prepare tables and graphs for written documents (papers or posters) first, and then re-use these figures in slides. However, slides have different considerations than written documents and there are different design principles to enhance communication and clarity.

	Before	**After**

Only include data in tables that you will actively show or discuss. Adding gridlines to tables in slide presentations is helpful for audiences who must examine data from a distance.

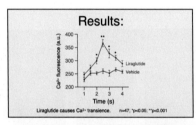

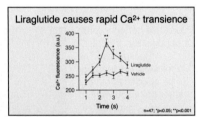

Place graph and table titles at the top of the slide and footnotes at the bottom. To help the audience perceive the meaning of data, the best title of a data slide states the overall result or conclusion.

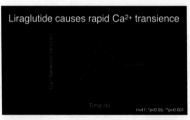

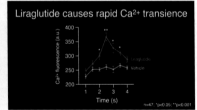

Ensure there is contrast between foreground and background. If a figure was originally made to stand out against a white background, you may need to invert the foreground colors for a darker slide.

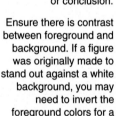

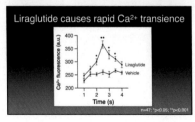

Audiences will have an easier time reading your data slides if you use the same background color as your tables and graphs. Try not to introduce unnecessary visual clutter.

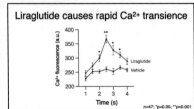

Try to only present one table or graph per slide

Audiences can only reflect meaningfully on one piece of information at a time. Therefore, try only to show one graph or figure per slide unless you have a good reason not to do so.

Before

After

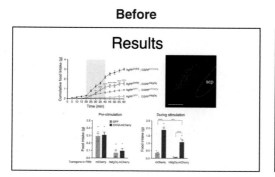

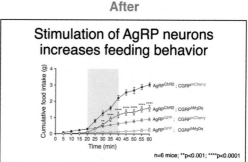

Although many presenters intend to discuss only one figure at a time, they nevertheless display multiple figures on the same slide, addressing each sequentially. The problem with this strategy is that each chart is much smaller than it needs to be, and also that audiences always break their focus and look at whatever figure catches their eye, no matter which figure the speaker is actively talking about.

If you want to present two or more figures side-by-side for comparison or discussion, consider presenting them individually at first and then grouping them together afterward.

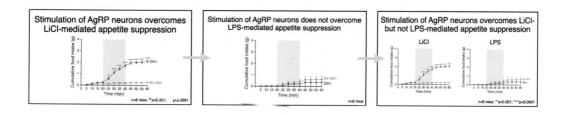

Animate data in tables and graphs for emphasis

One of the advantages of slide presentations compared with any other science presentation format is your ability to emphasize information in tables and graphs using simple entry/exit animation techniques. Doing so allows you to highlight specific datasets or even specific data points at a time of your choosing.

Animate the entrance of data to emphasize each category, one at a time.

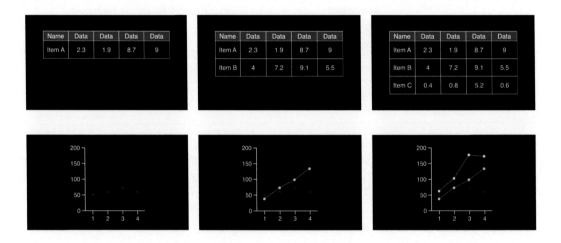

Animate with color and shapes to highlight individual data points.

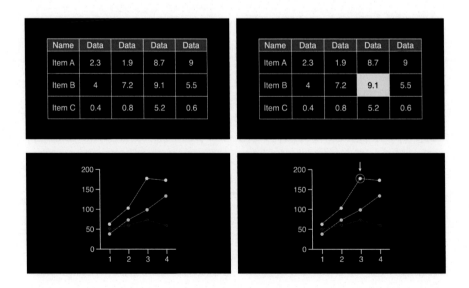

Optimize diagrams for slides

As discussed in Chapter 8, diagrams are useful when they have more explanatory power than words or photographs alone. In contrast with research articles and poster presentations, you can use as many explanatory diagrams as you would like in a slide presentation.

Diagrams are relatively easy to create in slide-making applications because of how simple it is to draw shapes, lines and arrows. In fact, many scientists create their diagrams in PowerPoint or Keynote and then export them for use in written or poster presentations.

As with any other presentation format, use design principles to optimize diagrams for slides.

Before **After**

Pay attention to default settings such as the fonts, colors, and thickness of lines. Deliberately adjust each until your diagram is optimal.

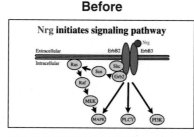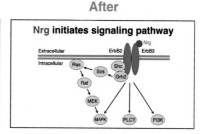

Avoid the temptation to fill each item with a different color. Use warm colors minimally, only to emphasize the most important aspect of your diagram.

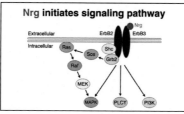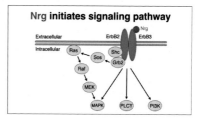

Like tables and graphs, another major advantage of slide presentations is the ability to animate diagrams to enhance communication with an audience.

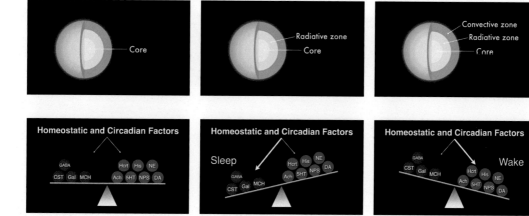

Optimize photographs for slides

Because slide presentations are not as formal or space-limited as written or poster presentations, they are an ideal medium for using photographs, both to show data and to visually communicate concepts to audiences.

Before | **After**

Photographs are much more engaging than text. Consider replacing long sections of text with a representative photograph that will instantly communicate a concept.

Water erosion can cause bite-like groves in metamorphic rock

- Metamorphic rocks are typically formed by the recrystallization of pre-existing rocks
- Rocks form under uniform pressure and heat
- After formation, softer rock can be cleared away by erosion in rivers and streams
- Grooves can sometimes take on bite-like appearances that resemble fossils

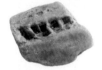

Water erosion can cause bite-like groves in metamorphic rock

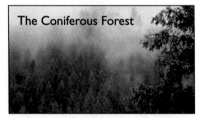

If your photograph is of a high enough resolution, consider increasing its impact by enlarging it to fill the entire slide.

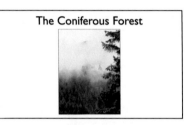
The Coniferous Forest

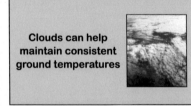
The Coniferous Forest

If a photograph is too small to fill the entire slide, place it within a minimal frame so that it stands out from the background.

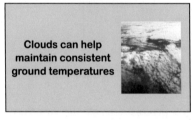
Clouds can help maintain consistent ground temperatures

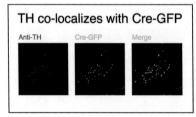
Clouds can help maintain consistent ground temperatures

When presenting fluorescent images, use a dark background so that the signal is the brightest aspect of the visual scene.

TH co-localizes with Cre-GFP

Anti-TH   Cre-GFP   Merge

TH co-localizes with Cre-GFP

Anti-TH   Cre-GFP   Merge

Before

After

The corpus callosum connects
the two halves of the brain

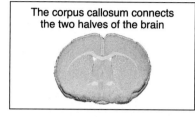

The corpus callosum connects
the two halves of the brain

Corpus
callosum

Make sure your audience knows what they are looking at. Explain a photograph, either through oral narration or by using subtle labels.

Surgical implants

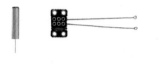

Surgical implants

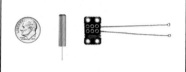

Sometimes it can be useful to include a reference for scale, so the audience intuitively understands the relative size of objects.

How does the
brain regulate
Thirst?

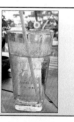

How does the
brain regulate
Thirst?

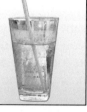

Consider extracting foreground objects in photos from their backgrounds to remove distractions and to increase the harmony with your slide background.

Natural sugars   **Refined sugars**

http://www.wafin.wa/product/apples-organic/   http://www.martinco/candy/f5sg5ge4lvgg44325gd

Natural sugars   **Refined sugars**

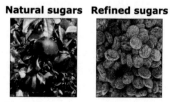

If you found images online, consider citing their sources all at once at the end of your presentation (with a "credits" slide) rather than including distracting or wordy citations within the slides themselves.

Optimize videos for slides

When appropriate, videos are one of the best tools you can add to a slide presentation. Not only do they dramatically show data or ideas in ways that static images or words alone cannot, they also function as something like an "audience reset button," immediately increasing attention and enthusiasm in anyone who may have lost focus. The moment a speaker says, "Let me play you a quick movie," every single audience member immediately looks attentively at the screen. It's like magic.

Only show videos when they help communicate data or ideas:

- Show a single trial of an experiment so your audience instantly understands your methods and procedures.

- Show the rotation of a three-dimensional object so your audience has a better perspective. For example, a three-dimensional rotation of the anatomy of an organ.

- Show a video that depicts changes that occur over time, such as an animated map of the United States that shows obesity trends over the past 50 years.

- Show a case study, such as a brief movie of a patient who suffers from a specific disease that you address in your presentation.

- Show a clip from a popular TV show or movie that helps illustrate a point—for example, a relevant news clip or joke from a late night program that addresses your research topic.

Add a video when relevant to your presentation, but also consider adding a quick clip during moments when you think your audience may need a break during a long stretch of technical information. Including a video can simultaneously communicate information, increase attention, and provide the audience with a mental break after a long stretch of data.

In addition to using your own movies, you can find many great movies to add to your science presentations by searching video sites such as YouTube. Many free websites exist that convert YouTube videos into presentation formats that you can embed into your presentation. Many of the best scientific movies can be found as supplementary videos in scientific papers. To find these movies, type the subject of your search plus the words "supplementary movie" into your favorite search engine.

Before   **After**

To avoid the time and interruption required to pause a slide show and play a movie file, try to embed a movie directly within a presentation.

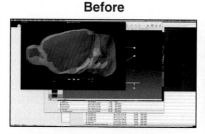 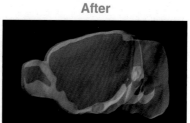

If the resolution is high enough, enlarge a video so that it fills the slide.

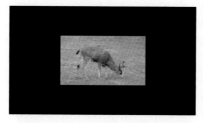 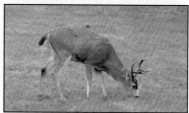

If your video doesn't have the resolution to fill the slide, ensure that it stands out from the background. Consider framing it within a subtle border.

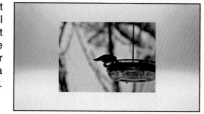 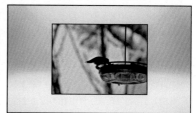

Add labels or animation on top of a video to help show your audience what is most important.

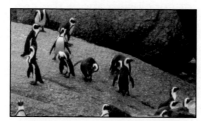 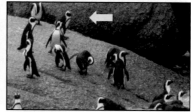

To immediately engage your audience as they enter the room, consider continuously playing a movie as part of a title slide. In this example, a video of rush hour in Vietnam immediately captures attention.

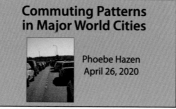 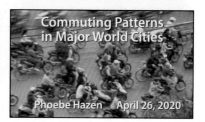

Summary: Design principles for visual elements in slides

- Because a typical presentation slide can only contain a few visual elements, the design choices you make about each will have a consequential impact on your ability to communicate with your audience.

- Avoid the temptation to add decoration to a slide to increase its esthetic value. Instead of decoration, add good design choices. Well-designed slides will look beautiful as a consequence and better convey information to an audience.

- Before designing a presentation, find out if the presentation venue is optimized for standard (4:3) versus widescreen (16:9) slides. While it is possible to present a presentation in either format, optimizing your slides for the given format will allow you to make better choices about slide sizes and layout.

- Choose inconspicuous backgrounds for slides that won't distract from the much more important foreground content. Optimize the contrast between your foregrounds and backgrounds so that visual information is easy to see.

- Choose colors for backgrounds and foregrounds judiciously, using color sparingly to highlight important information.

- Choose fonts that are legible throughout the presentation room.

- Audiences don't like to read long stretches of text, so keep text on slides to a minimum. Likewise, minimize the use of long lists and outlines.

- Use slide titles to make a point or conclusion about the contents of a slide.

- Optimize tables and graphs for slides so that they are easy to see and read across a presentation room. Try to only present one table or graph per slide so the audience only needs to keep track of one piece of information at a time.

- Consider animating individual aspects of tables and graphs to show your audience key pieces of information when you are ready to explain them.

- Optimize diagrams and photographs for slides to decrease the amount of time required to perceive and understand information.

- Optimize videos for slides to better communicate videos and ideas, and also to deliberately capture an audience's attention.

16

Slide layout

Slide layout refers to how you arrange visual elements on a slide. When arranging the figures for a written manuscript or designing the layout of a scientific poster, you have some flexibility in how you arrange visual information, but are also constrained by the traditional structure of these formats. In contrast, when designing a slide presentation, you have greater freedom to arrange visual elements however you want. Slide layout has a tremendous impact on your ability to communicate information to an audience. An optimal layout imparts a flow of information, establishes a hierarchy of what is most important, and creates harmonious relationships among distinct visual elements. Therefore, good slide layout allows the impact of a slide to be much more than the sum of its parts.

Designing Science Presentations. https://doi.org/10.1016/B978-0-12-815377-2.00016-0

Be deliberate about slide layout to tell a better visual story

In addition to optimizing individual visual elements, designing a slide requires arranging these elements in a logical way to help the audience perceive and process information.

Arranging visual elements on a slide is much more consequential than simply making a slide "look nice." Slide layout is about controlling the flow of information, emphasizing what is most important, and establishing relationships between different visual elements.

When a scientist creates a slide without designing an optimal layout, the meaning of visual elements can become obscured, and the slides themselves can seem overwhelming, random, and yes, even ugly.

Slides that could use a good layout tune-up:

Too busy and overwhelming

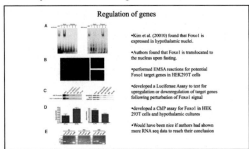

Too random

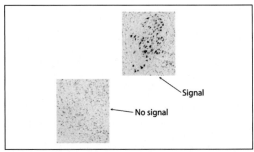

Too sparse and assymetric

Too loud and complex

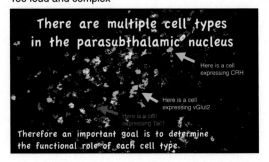

To be deliberate about slide layout, avoid universal slide templates

All slide making applications are packaged with several slide templates—master slides with a prearranged layout that users can fill with their own content. These master slides can be useful for anyone new to creating slide shows because they quickly teach novices how to add and arrange content on a slide.

The problem with templates is that they are not specific to your own content. The software engineers who created these templates deliberately designed them to be universal and applicable to most kinds of visual information. Although these templates may present your content adequately, they are certainly not designed to communicate specific messages optimally.

Instead of using templates, start with a blank canvas and intentionally lay out your content in the way that best communicates your message.

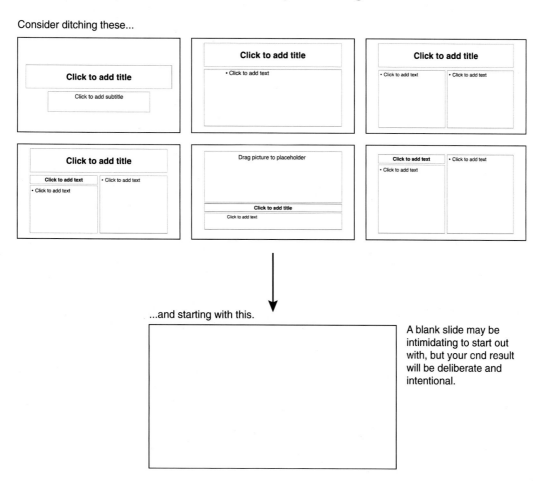

Consider ditching these...

...and starting with this.

A blank slide may be intimidating to start out with, but your end result will be deliberate and intentional.

Design a natural flow of information

Each time you advance to a new slide in your presentation, your audience immediately begins scanning the slide for information. Help them out by designing a natural, visually intuitive order of information.

Audiences have a natural tendency to read a slide as they would a book. In Western cultures, we start by gazing from the top left to top right and finish by gazing from the bottom left to bottom right. Therefore, to provide your audience with an intuitive flow of information, try laying out your content with this paradigm in mind.

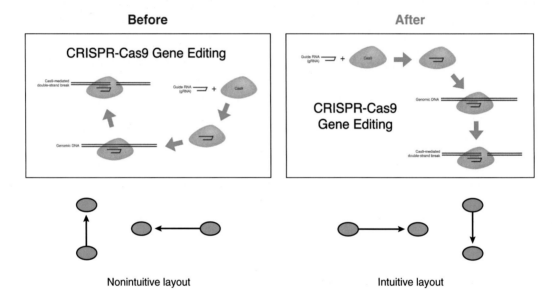

Without thinking about it, audiences should know immediately whether information is grouped in rows or columns.

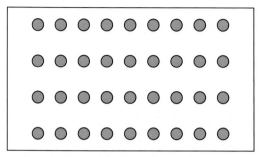

Audiences will process information grouped into rows by reading each row left to right and descending top to bottom.

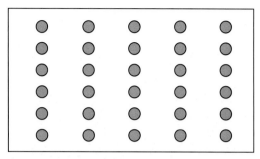

Audiences will process information grouped into columns by reading each column top to bottom and proceeding left to right.

If it is necessary to organize the flow of visual information in a way that is different from a natural reading style, guide the audience with arrows or by varying the size of visual elements.

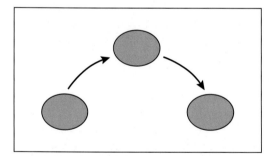

Arrows immediately convey the proper flow of information to an audience. However, even if you use arrows, try to organize information from left to right or top to bottom to create a natural reading experience.

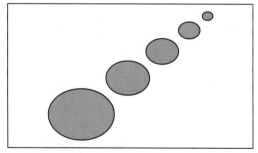

In the absence of arrows or other visual cues, audiences tend to perceive bigger objects as the foreground and will scan visual elements from largest to smallest.

Emphasize important visual elements

Just as with diagrams, it is possible to emphasize visual elements within a slide by varying simple parameters.

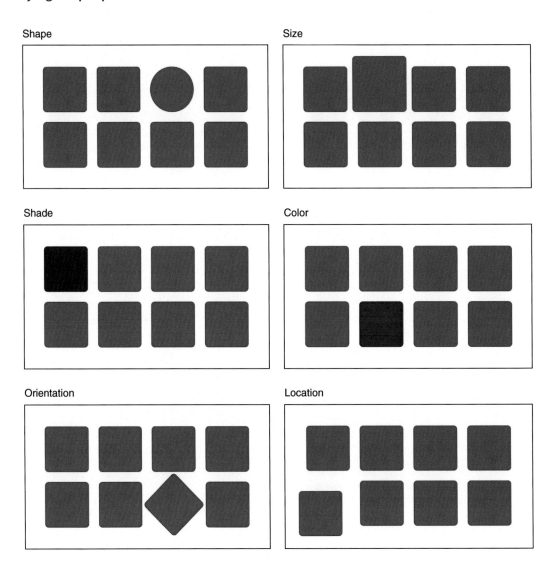

Each time you arrange elements on a slide, you make a statement about their relative importance. Even if you don't explicitly state what you find most important, the audience will make conclusions about what you are trying to emphasize based on your slide layout. Therefore, be deliberate about arranging your elements so that your most crucial information is emphasized the most.

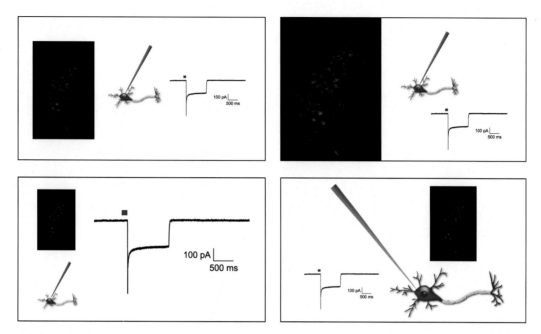

All of these slides present the same figures but emphasize them differently based on size and location. Each slide makes a different statement about which figure is most important.

Align visual elements for harmony

The human eye is remarkably good at perceiving the proper alignment of visual elements. When objects are not aligned, it can take longer for audiences to perceive the meaning of visual information and slides are not as pleasing to look at.

In contrast, when visual elements are aligned evenly on a slide, your arrangement conveys a sense of order and harmony. Your audience members might not be consciously aware of this harmony, but they will pay more attention to your presentation because your slides will be more pleasing to view.

Before **After**

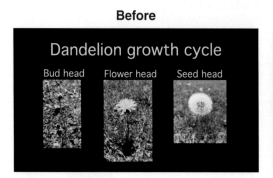 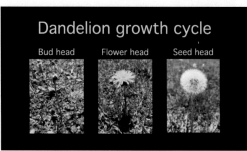

In the slide on the left, the three images are slightly disjointed and not evenly spaced. The labels above the images are not aligned and sometimes spill off the edge on the right side. The slide on the right is much more balanced because the image sizes have been adjusted to the same width and height. Additionally, the labels are all centered above the images.

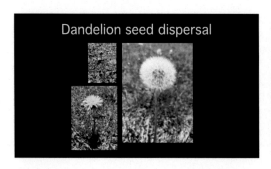 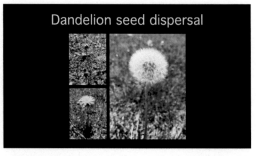

In the slide on the left, the bottom left image stands out even though the right image is much larger. If this is intentional, kudos to the author for using design principles to deliberately emphasize the bottom left image. However, if this is unintentional, adjust the widths and heights of the images until the entire visual scene achieves a sense of balance.

Align visual elements using a grid

When arranging elements on a slide, it can be helpful to imagine an invisible grid (or you can use a grid included in your slide making application) to aid in good alignment. A grid with three rows and three columns follows the principle of the "rule of thirds" (see Chapter 9). Aligning objects along these lines or at their intersections creates a harmonious scene with a remarkable simplicity. In addition to the rule of thirds, you can design a grid with however many rows and columns as you would like. In slides, creating a 4 × 3 or 4 × 4 grid can also achieve excellent results.

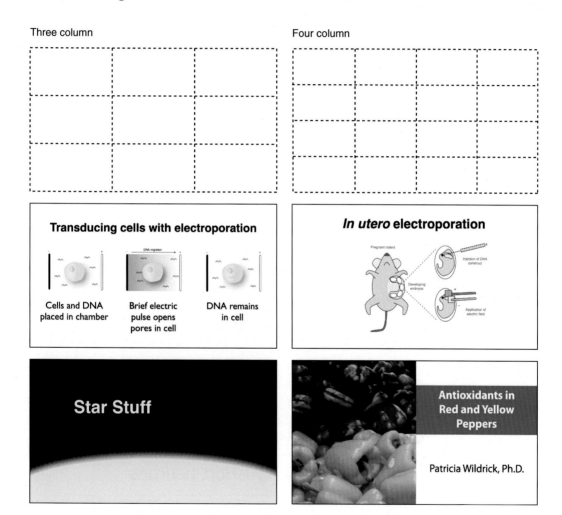

Embrace simplicity

Visual elements on slides are like people in an elevator: you can theoretically fit a maximum capacity into a tiny space, but it's nice to have some breathing room.

People new to making slide presentations often feel the need to fill their slides with too many visual elements. In reality, the old maxim "less is more" truly holds for slides. Putting less on a slide adds greater impact to the information that you choose to show, increasing the clarity of your message and simplicity of your delivery.

Before

After

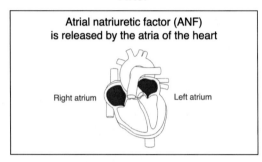

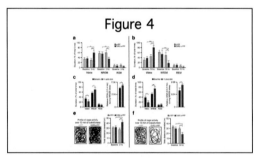

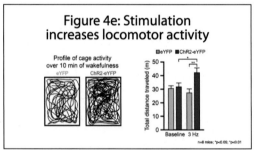

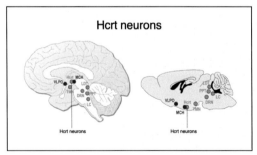

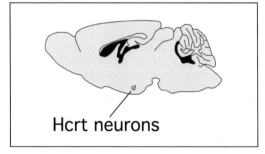

Split busy slides into multiple slides

The best slides are clear, simple, and only convey a single idea. If you find yourself creating a slide that contains too much information (such as a slide with several bullet points), consider splitting your slide into three to five separate slides.

Don't believe the myth that each slide takes a minute to present ... in reality, it will probably take you less time to present five ideas on five slides compared with five ideas on one slide because your presentation will be more clear and easier for your audience to understand.

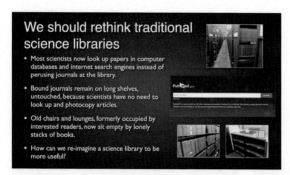

This slide contains multiple ideas and images. As the speaker explains each bullet point, this single, busy slide remains projected in the background. Instead, why not present the same information as a series of separate slides, each with its own message?

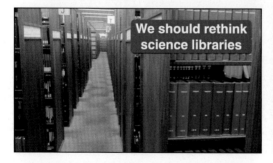

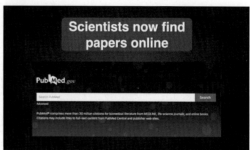

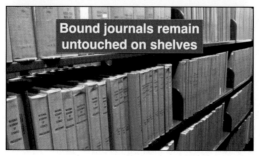

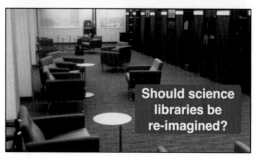

Achieve harmony with photographs

When including photos of dynamic or conscious subjects, it is pleasing to an audience to incorporate the subjects as part of the overall visual scene of a slide. Subjects that seem to be moving or staring away from your visual scene can disrupt the harmony of your slide and distract from your message. Use simple photo flipping or rotating techniques to make sure that all of your visual elements are congruent with each other.

Before

After

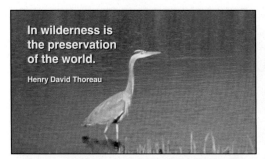
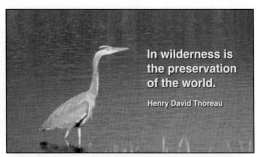
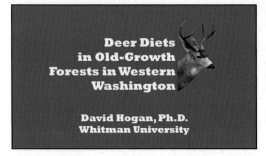
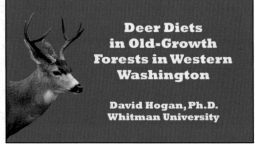

Summary: Design principles for slide layout

- Slide layout refers to how you arrange visual elements on a slide to achieve an optimal flow of information, hierarchy of what is most important, and overall harmony.

- Avoid universal slide templates or master slides that suggest where to place objects. Instead, start with a blank canvas and intentionally layout your content in the way that best communicates your message.

- Design a natural flow of information so that your audience knows what to look at first, second, third, etc.

- Emphasize important visual elements by varying their shape, size, shade, color, orientation, or location.

- Align visual elements on a slide to achieve a balanced, harmonious quality that will make your slides more pleasing to view.

- Embrace simplicity, and allow visual elements within a slide some breathing room. If there are too many elements on one slide, consider splitting busy slides into multiple slides.

- When including photos of dynamic or conscious subjects, incorporate these subjects into the visual scene of a slide as much as possible.

17

Slide animations and transitions

Slide animation effects allow you to make visual elements appear, disappear, and move around the screen. Transition effects allow you to advance from one slide to the next with a variety of two- and three-dimensional effects. These effects are usually fun to play with and generally look exciting when you first see them. However, from a design point of view, we should always ask what benefit these effects add to a presentation. When are they useful and when are they decorative? When do they add clarity and when do they add distraction? As with all other presentation tools, animation and transition effects can add great value if used for a meaningful purpose.

Designing Science Presentations. https://doi.org/10.1016/B978-0-12-815377-2.00017-2

The benefits of using slide animation effects

Animation and transition effects are a wonderful feature of slide presentation applications that did not exist with classic manual slide projectors. Before PowerPoint, Keynote, and Google Slides, photographic slide projectors could only display static visual scenes. The only way that a presenter could add an animation effect was to advance to a slightly different slide, which was cost-prohibitive because each slide was expensive to produce. Modern slide applications allow for many kinds of animation techniques that can increase your ability to communicate complex information to an audience.

There are many reasons why it might be beneficial to add animation to a slide presentation:

- To make visual elements appear only when you want your audience to see them

- To remove visual elements when they are no longer relevant to your message

- To direct an audience's visual attention

- To increase understanding about how a process works by showing how individual components dynamically interact

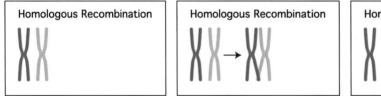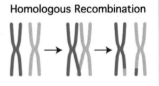

One of the benefits of using animation techniques is the ability to control the flow of information. Audience members see what you want them to see, *when* you want them to see it.

Don't use animation effects when they don't add value or information. For example, if presenting an image of a pipette injecting liquid into a solution, would it add value to animate liquid dispensing from the pipette tip? Do you want your audience's attention focused on the pipette, or on the information you are trying to communicate? Effects that don't add meaning are a potential distraction to your audience and a potential waste of time to create.

Don't be an animation show-off

Using animation effects in presentations is a feature that can easily be abused. When creating slides, it can be fun to explore the animation tricks at your disposal and play with cool special effects; however, during an actual presentation, make sure that these effects actually add value to your ability to communicate information to your audience.

Remember that good design never calls attention to itself. Presentation effects should always be used in service of your science and not in service of the cool tricks you know how to perform with your computer.

Although the slide software you use may provide you with the power to bounce text around your slide, turn your diagrams into smoke, or explode photographs into a burst of flame, always ask yourself whether such techniques add value to your presentation. Days after your talk is over, will your audience remember your three-dimensional explosion effects or will they remember you and the information you shared?

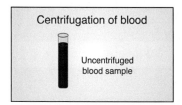 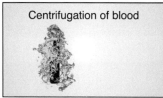 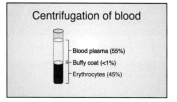

In this series of slides, a speaker animates the transition between two diagrams with an explosion effect. Although this explosion animation may look cool, it does not add value. Psychologically, it is strange to combine the concepts of blood samples and fire. The audience may smile and appear impressed, but they will likely be distracted from the main scientific message.

Use animation to introduce concepts at a time of your choosing

One of the advantages of slide shows compared with other presentation formats is the ability to show whatever you want, whenever you want. Animation effects let you precisely control when your audience will see specific visual elements.

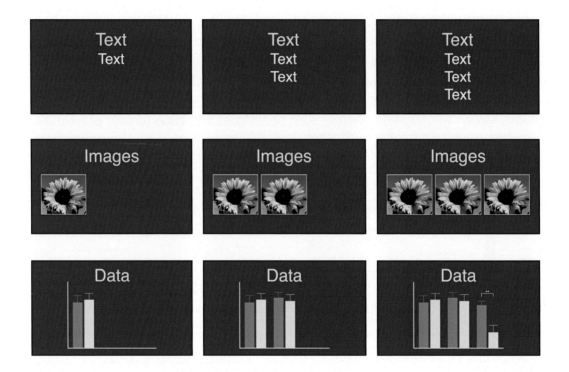

Keep in mind that when a single visual element appears in the top or left-hand side of the screen, your audience is primed to expect more. Therefore, don't keep them in suspense for long. If you are too slow to introduce subsequent text or images, your audience will become impatient or distracted.

Use animation to relate the big and the small

Using "scale" or "zoom" animation features, you can make visual elements much bigger or smaller during your presentation. These techniques are useful for showing how an object might literally shrink or enlarge during a process—for example, in a slide about how a star expands as it grows old. Additionally, you can scale an object to demonstrate how an individual component of a system relates to a larger whole. In doing so, you can focus on a constituent part of a process while also showing a larger, global perspective.

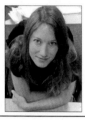 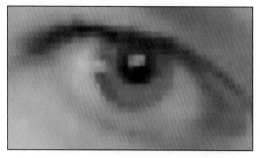

In this slide, a magnification animation effect is applied to the photograph until the eye fills the entire screen. This has a powerful effect, not only because the subject matter is about the human eye, but also because it is a perfect demonstration of the fact that the pixellated photograph on the right looks perfectly clear in a normally-sized photo, demonstrating to everyone the limitations of their own eyes.

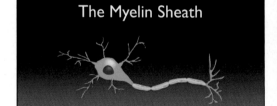 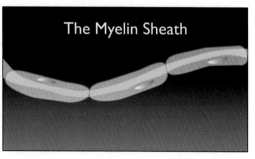

This slide starts with a global pictorial diagram of a neuron before zooming in to focus on the myelin sheath. The advantage of starting out with an entire neuron is that the audience conceptuallizes the complete object, always remembering that the specific component under investigation is part of a larger whole. At the end of the talk, the speaker could scale back down to remind the audience of the bigger picture.

Animate movements naturally and intuitively

Animation techniques are great for showing movement and how objects interact with each other.

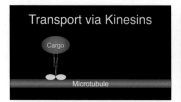 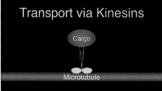 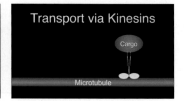

A simple animation effect moves cartoon biomolecules from left to right across a depiction of a microtubule. Instead of animating this movement quickly, a presenter could adjust the settings to move the object over a period of 30-40 seconds while they orally narrate the phenomenon.

If you apply movement to visual elements on your slide, animate them in a direction that is natural and intuitive to your audience. Otherwise, your animations may not resonate as effectively.

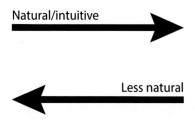

Because of how we are used to reading, it is more comfortable to experience movement going from left to right than right to left.

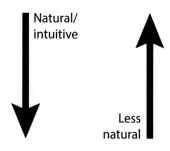

Because of our intuition of gravity, it is usually more comfortable to watch objects descend than rise.

Animate diagrams to bring dynamic processes to life

A good static diagram can quickly inform an audience about the steps in a process or technological procedure. Simple animations can add meaning and visual impact to these diagrams, bringing processes to life in a way that static diagrams cannot.

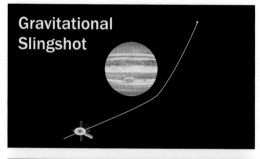

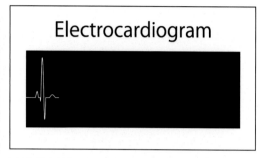

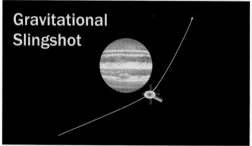

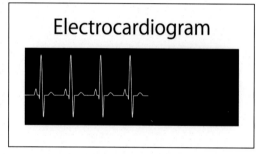

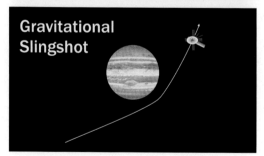

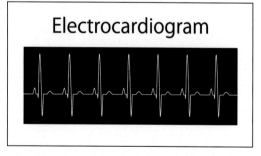

This slide conveys the gravitational assist experienced by a space probe passing a planet. In the animation, the probe approaches Jupiter, then the animation speeds up to demonstrate the increase in velocity.

This slide presents an animated electrocardiogram (ECG). A black rectangle is placed in front of an ECG trace, and a simple "wipe" animation removes the black to create the illusion of a real-time ECG recording. This animation can be looped continuously as the presenter conveys information orally. If used for no reason, such an animation could be distracting; however, in this case, the presenter might want to recreate the impression of observing a real-time recording in a clinical setting.

Use animation to direct the audience's attention

When the human eye perceives motion within a static visual scene, it immediately focuses on the moving object. Therefore, one way to direct an audience's attention to a particularly important feature is to animate the visual element with a brief subtle motion. This animation can be applied to a visual element as it appears on a slide, or to an object already present on a slide.

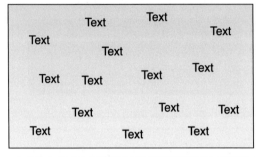
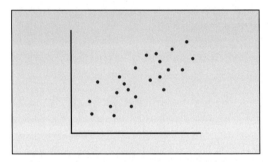
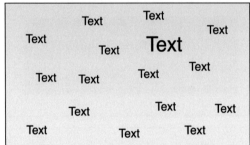
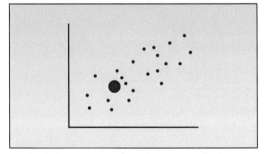
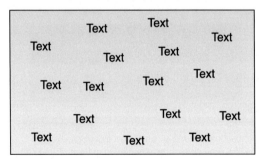
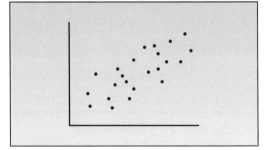

To introduce text or another visual element to a slide that already has many visual elements, use a pop or scaling effect so that the new object is momentarily visually salient.

To highlight a visual element among many other elements, briefly "pulse" the object in size as you describe the object's meaning.

Use slide transitions minimally for emphasis

The default slide transition setting in PowerPoint, Keynote, and Google Slides simply takes you from one slide to the next. These transitions, along with other peaceful effects like "fade in/out," are usually never consciously perceived by an audience.

However, these applications come bundled with a variety of exciting two- or three-dimensional transition effects that, while fun to look at, have the potential to divert your audience's attention. Like animating objects within slides, transitions should never distract from your main point. People who use gimmicky effects for each transition risk distracting their audience every time they advance to the next slide.

Be careful about using slide presentation software that is based entirely on gimmicky transition effects between slides. They are fun to play with, but their selling point is that the animations and transitions are exciting, not that your content will be the main attraction.

A benefit of more complicated transition effects is that, when used sparingly, they can refocus audience attention toward the screen. Like video, the movement of a slide transition causes your audience to look at the screen, even if only for a moment. If you use these effects constantly, your audience will stop attending to them; however, if only used three to five times during a presentation, they can be terrific tools to non-verbally inform your audience that you are transitioning from one major section of a talk to another. Chapter 14 suggested dividing the sections of a scientific talk into discrete segments of data. Perhaps the best occasion to use a transition effect is immediately before a new section of your talk. By momentarily regaining your audience's visual attention, you establish a new opportunity to engage them in your presentation.

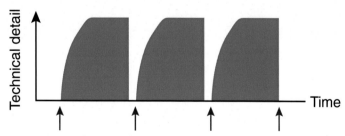

Potentially good moments for an animated slide transition

Use transitions to create scenes and panoramas

Slide transitions can be used as more than just a cute way to get from one slide to the next. Using the "push" transition, you can actually create impactful scenes that create the illusion of extending one slide into a longer landscape.

When using this technique, make sure to keep your slides as simple as possible and remove any background images, logos, slide numbers, etc. Adjust the settings so that each push lasts about 2–3 s.

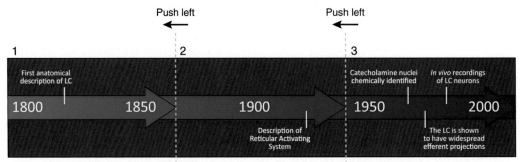

This series of three slides presents a 200-year timeline of the history of the study of a biological structure.

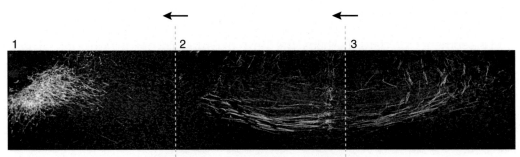

This series of three slides starts with a group of neurons and follows their projections across a brain.

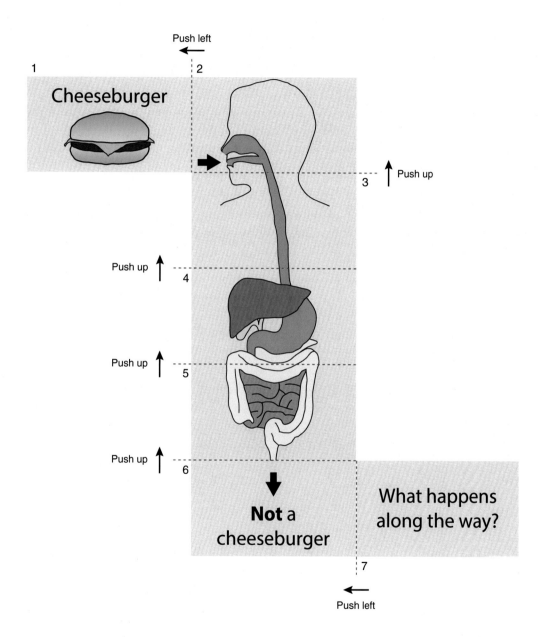

Summary: Design principles for slide animations and transitions

- Use slide animation and transition effects to help communicate information, not to add gimmicky effects just because they look cool.

- When using an animation or transition effect, ask yourself whether it helps you explain a concept or whether it potentially distracts from your explanation.

- Animation effects can be great tools for introducing concepts one at a time, for relating individual components of a system to a larger whole, for showing how objects move and interact with each other, and for purposefully directing the audience's attention to a salient visual element on a slide.

- Use slide transitions to refocus an audience's attention. The less you use slide transition effects, the more impactful they will be.

- Consider using slide transition effects to create larger scenes and panoramas (if they are helpful) that would be bigger than a single slide to display.

18

Delivering a slide presentation

After investing time and effort in designing a slide presentation, the final step is to prepare your delivery for an audience. Delivering a slide presentation often causes some anxiety. We don't want to come across as naïve, unsophisticated, or unskilled, and we are sometimes worried that our results will be unimpressive. At the same time, we want to wow an audience, impressing them not only with our data, but with a captivating delivery and command of the field. We might also hope to come across as charismatic, charming, and wise. Fortunately, the hallmarks of a great delivery have more to do with preparation than with the quality of our data or personality traits. It is possible to design the delivery of a presentation just as it is possible to design the story and slides. If you spent time preparing a great slide presentation, then you can complement that hard work by preparing and rehearsing an excellent delivery.

Designing Science Presentations. https://doi.org/10.1016/B978-0-12-815377-2.00018-4

To seem like a natural, design and rehearse

Every now and then, you will come across a scientific speaker who makes delivering an excellent talk seem effortless and natural. These speakers communicate complicated messages to audiences in a way that captivates everyone in the room, yet they look like they are hardly working at all. In reality, these speakers spend much time and effort to deliver a great talk, and much of the effectiveness of their delivery comes from substantial preparation.

What distinguishes "naturals" from others is the degree to which they design and rehearse talks until they communicate their message as effectively as possible. Ironically, the more a person prepares and rehearses, the more effortless and natural they seem.

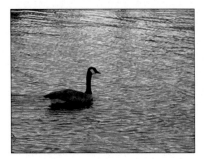

A great presenter is like a quintessential bird on the water: going from point to point seems effortless and graceful, yet beneath the surface, a great deal of work is required to stay afloat and push ahead.

Yes, some people are naturally more charismatic and animated than others, however, these traits are neither necessary nor sufficient for a great presentation. If you invested the effort to design a great presentation for your audience, including both a logical flow of information and well-designed, visually accessible slides, then you have already completed most of the work of delivering a great presentation. All you need to do now is prepare and rehearse your delivery to ensure the most effective talk possible.

How best to rehearse? The truth is that everyone rehearses differently. Some like to rehearse by actually delivering their talks in a presentation room, but don't feel this is the only way to rehearse if it makes you feel awkward or uncomfortable. Some people rehearse best mentally: at their desks, on a walk, in the shower, etc. Rehearse in whatever way best allows you to practice what you will say to your audience.

Strategies for dealing with anxiety

Most speakers experience anxiety about presentation delivery, especially in the moments leading up to the start of their talks. Anxiety occurs in speakers at all career levels, even in scientists who have a reputation for giving great talks. In fact, a presenter who seems the most comfortable when presenting might actually be the most nervous of all!

Don't let presentation anxiety interfere with your ability to deliver a great presentation. Practice and preparation distinguish presenters who don't seem nervous from presenters who let anxiety overcome their delivery.

If you anticipate being nervous before your talk, prepare by developing strategies to transform anxiety into positive energy:

Rehearse for the 5 min before your presentation begins. Speakers usually become the most nervous just before their talks begin. To prepare, anticipate the sights and sounds of the minutes just before your talk, especially the sounds of a gathering audience. In fact … the next time you attend a talk, record 5—10 min of audience chatter on your phone—if you listen to these sounds as you prepare for a talk, you will become accustomed to them and feel less nervous!

Memorize and meticulously rehearse the first 1—2 min of your talk. Most speakers agree that once they get through the first minute of their presentation, anxiety begins to fade. Therefore, memorize and rehearse the first 1—2 min so that you feel more in control at the very beginning and you are guaranteed to make a great first impression.

Become comfortable around your presentation space. To the degree to which it is possible, become familiar and comfortable with your presentation space. If your talk will take place at your institution, spend some time standing where you will stand during the actual talk to make yourself feel more at home. If you are traveling, try to take a brief moment before or after setting up just to reflect on where you are and the environment around you. Feeling comfortable in your presentation space will go a long way toward making you feel comfortable in general.

Consider walking throughout your presentation space during your talk. Although it is tempting to hide behind a lectern, slowly walking around your available presentation space will help calm anxiety and also give you the perception that you are having a friendly conversation with your audience. Use a remote slide advancer (see Chapter 19) so that you are free to leave your computer and speak from wherever you feel most comfortable.

Bring a water bottle. Presentation anxiety can often cause a dry mouth due to the physiological response to stress. It's always nice to have a water bottle with you. You might not need it, but you'll be glad you can take a quick sip if you do!

Place yourself front and center

The audience members attending your scientific talk don't only want to see your slides, they want to see and hear *you*. Strive to be fully visible and audible to your audience, and to fully engage them with your presence and voice. By increasing the degree to which your audience can see and hear you throughout your talk, you increase the passion you convey as well as the likelihood that your audience will pay attention.

To increase your presence and ability to engage with an audience:

Leave the lights on: Never turn the lights off all the way unless you need to temporarily shut them off for a specific slide (e.g., a fluorescent microscopy image).

Make sure your voice projects throughout the room: Do a quick sound check before the start of your talk. If delivering in a large room, practice using the microphone to ensure that your voice is effortlessly heard throughout the entire room without booming.

Try not to sit behind a table or lectern: If possible, use a remote slide advancer so that you can leave your computer and walk around the entire presentation space. If it is necessary to stand at a podium, a remote slide advancer gives you freedom to stand from side to side and not be confined to standing directly in front of your computer.

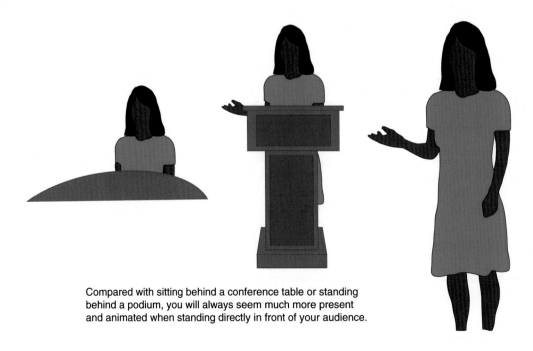

Compared with sitting behind a conference table or standing behind a podium, you will always seem much more present and animated when standing directly in front of your audience.

Immediately gain rapport with your audience

You can establish an immediate emotional connection with your audience members by addressing them specifically at the start of your talk, commenting on what you appreciate about them, how they are likely to feel, or what they are likely to want to hear from you. By addressing your audience members directly, you form an instant relationship with your audience that causes them to not only be invested in your talk but also with you.

Comment on who they are:

It is a real pleasure to be speaking at the University of Washington again. I always love visiting here because you have so many of the world's best behavioral neuroscientists all in the same place. It has been a true pleasure to meet with so many of you throughout the day and I hope to visit with more of you after my talk.

Thank you for inviting me to speak at your lab meeting! Obviously, we are interested in similar topics and this lab has inspired many of the experiments I performed in the past. This is a great opportunity for me to share what I've been working on lately and get your feedback, and it would be great if any collaborations develop because of our mutual interests.

Comment on how they are likely to feel:

First of all, thank you very much for attending my talk at 8:00 in the morning ... especially on the fourth day of a 4-day conference. I know some of you were up late last night because, well, frankly, I was with some of you. So I know many of you are tired and I'm so appreciative you woke up to be here. I promise to make it worth your while.

How are you guys holding up? I know it's the middle of midterm season and I hear that anyone taking general chemistry or organic chemistry just had a big exam yesterday. You must be tired. Let's try to put that stress aside for a moment to talk about something fun.

Comment on what they are likely to want to hear from you:

I picked this journal club paper not only because it is a great paper, but because the authors addressed a scientific problem that is similar to a lot of the problems we address in our lab. I think that the strategies that these authors used could be potentially adapted by many of you to achieve your own goals.

I'm sure that you not only came to hear my talk because of my own research topic, but because you might also be interested in doing experiments with copper-based nanotubules. Today, in addition to talking about my own work, I'll be sure to talk about the development and application of these tools so that you can apply them to your own work.

Aim to be present

You have probably attended scientific talks in which the speaker seemed to lack an accurate impression of how the talk was going. Whether because of something the speaker was doing, the audience's level of enthusiasm or comprehension, or even something about the presentation room itself, some aspect of the talk wasn't ideal, and the speaker failed to accurately gauge the atmosphere.

Part of the skill of delivering a talk is to be fully in the moment, and to continuously monitor your communication during the actual delivery.

To be present as a speaker means to have a clear understanding of yourself, your audience, and your environment during your real-time delivery.

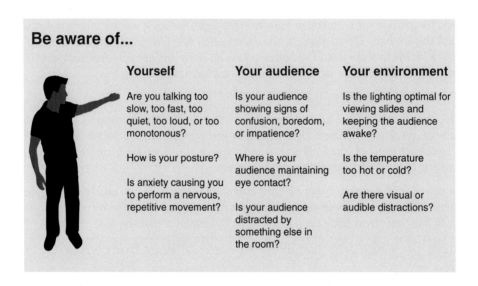

Be aware of...

Yourself	Your audience	Your environment
Are you talking too slow, too fast, too quiet, too loud, or too monotonous?	Is your audience showing signs of confusion, boredom, or impatience?	Is the lighting optimal for viewing slides and keeping the audience awake?
How is your posture?	Where is your audience maintaining eye contact?	Is the temperature too hot or cold?
Is anxiety causing you to perform a nervous, repetitive movement?	Is your audience distracted by something else in the room?	Are there visual or audible distractions?

Being present is a true skill that requires active practice and experience. Each time you give a talk, train yourself to occasionally gauge your speaking style, to look for the attentiveness of the audience, or to address any distractions in the environment. The more often you practice being in the moment, the more likely you will be to develop good monitoring habits for future talks.

Don't use slides as presentation notes

Consciously or unconsciously, many scientists add text to their slides to help them remember what to say during their delivery. It can be comforting to know that all of the information you want to communicate is immediately available to you, however, there are a number of disadvantages. Slides with too much text are visually unappealing and much less likely to resonate with audiences. If you look at the slides rather than maintaining eye contact with your audience, you will lose the ability to address your audience directly. Finally, looking at slides reduces your ability to be present and attentive to the real-time needs and reactions of your audience.

Ask yourself whether the text on your slides is for your audience's benefit or for your own. Remember that slides should primarily serve as a visual aid, not a page of notes.

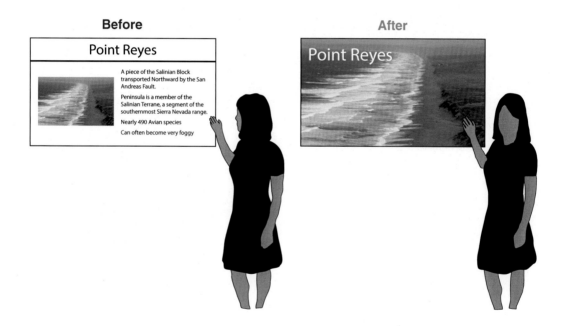

Rehearse to the point at which you no longer need presentation notes. If necessary, bring a very brief page of key points in case you want to refer to some quick facts.

Work toward eliminating verbal distractions

Just as it is beneficial to remove clutter from your slides that doesn't add value, it is also beneficial to eliminate wordiness from your oral delivery that doesn't help communicate information to an audience. Verbal distractions can interrupt the flow of your presentation and also waste valuable time.

Everyone is prone to their own verbal distractions, but some are more common than others.

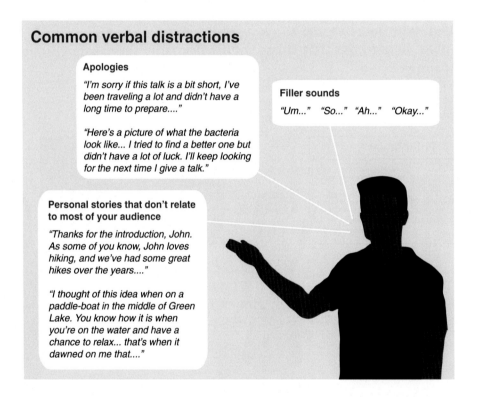

Sometimes presentation anxiety causes you to say things you don't intend. While in the moment of presenting, people can be unconscious to their own verbal hiccups. If you find yourself succumbing to one of the verbal distractions above, you can eliminate these habits with practice. Each time you present a talk, try to consciously focus on extinguishing a particular bad habit. Over time and with practice, these verbal distractions will disappear.

Strategies for answering audience questions

Most scientific talks usually end with an opportunity for members of the audience to ask questions. Although this period might cause anxiety, make it a habit to smile and seem receptive to all questions. Your projected sense of calm and ease will convey confidence and inspire an atmosphere of collegiality and good will.

After receiving a question, consider briefly rephrasing the question in your own words before providing an answer. Doing so not only ensures that everyone in the audience hears and understands a question, but also that you correctly interpreted the specific question asked.

It is okay to not know the answer to a question. Most scientific fields are complicated both in terms of factual information and in terms of the literature. Therefore, feel free to admit the limits of your knowledge and to speculate on answers you don't know.

Although most audience members ask questions with good intentions, some questions can be more pointed and distracting than others. These questions commonly show up in a few different forms:

Overly critical questions: Although healthy skepticism and critical feedback is important in science, some audience members may ask questions that come across as overly critical and negative in tone. Perhaps the best approach is to acknowledge that the question addresses a valid concern, to answer as best as you can at the time, and to offer to discuss aspects of your science after the talk is over.

Time consuming questions: Sometimes a single audience member will monopolize the question and answer period with a long comment or stretch of questions. The best approach for dealing with a time-consuming question is to politely absorb the responsibility by suggesting that it will take *you* a long time for a meaningful answer, and to suggest a longer conversation after the talk.

Rudimentary questions: Although there really is no such thing as a dumb question, every now and then an audience member unfamiliar with your field may ask a question that isn't focused on your research, but focused on the fundamental underlying principles that most of the audience is already likely to know. Again, the best approach is to offer to talk after the question and answer session is over. "I can tell you a lot about that .... How about we talk in much more detail at the reception."

Summary: Design principles for delivering slide presentations

- If you have invested time and effort in designing a great slide presentation, much of the work of delivering the presentation is already completed. The final step is to practice what you will say during the actual delivery.

- To come across as a naturally great presenter actually requires much time preparing and rehearsing your delivery. Ironically, the more a person rehearses, the more effortless and natural they will seem.

- Many speakers across career levels experience anxiety about presenting in front of others. If you become anxious before talks, develop strategies for transforming anxiety into positive energy.

- Increase your presence and ability to engage with an audience by ensuring you are fully visible and audible throughout the presentation room.

- Gain rapport with an audience at the start of your presentation by addressing them directly, either about who they are, how they are likely to feel, or what they might hope to hear from you.

- Aim to be fully in the moment during a talk, continuously monitoring your speaking style, the level of attentiveness or comprehension of the audience, or potential distractions in the environment.

- Don't use slides as presentation notes because they will limit your ability to fully engage with your audience.

- Over time, work toward reducing the verbal clutter in the words you say to an audience. Many of these verbal distractions come from anxiety, but can be fixed over time.

- Develop skills for answering audience questions. Try to always smile and remain engaged with an audience during the question and answer period, and develop strategies for dealing with overly negative or distracting questions.

19

Using technology to present like a professional

Imagine a scientist who spends time and effort designing a beautiful presentation, and rehearses to ensure a fluid delivery. However, when it is time to present, they have a difficult time connecting their laptop to a projector because they don't have the right adapter. During the talk, slides appear too dark and fluorescent images are barely perceptible. The scientist tries to turn down the lights, but can't find the correct switch. Although the audience members understand the content, they are distracted by each technological mishap, and the scientist comes across as not being in control. Audiences associate good presentation technology skills with good presentation skills in general. Therefore, mastering presentation technology is the final step in delivering a great science presentation.

Designing Science Presentations. https://doi.org/10.1016/B978-0-12-815377-2.00019-6

Bring your own power and projection cords

Every computer comes with its own cord for connecting to a power outlet, and many, especially Macs, have unique cords for connecting to a digital projector. If you plan on using your laptop during a talk, you should consider it your responsibility to bring your own cords to the presentation venue. You don't want to have to ask around for a cord in the moments before your talk begins.

It is unlikely that someone will have the particular cords and adapters for your particular laptop. Bring your own cords so you don't have to nervously find one in the moments before your talk.

Almost all projectors connect to a computer via a 15-pin VGA connector or (especially in newer projectors) an HDMI connector. Therefore, your laptop should have a port to connect to a VGA or HDMI connection cable, or you should have an adapter that connects your computer to one of these ports.

VGA   HDMI

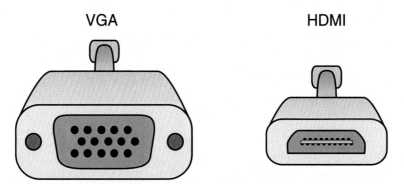

To connect to a projector, your laptop ports or your adaptors must contain a "female" receiving end for a 15-pin VGA cable (left) or for an HDMI cable (right). Newer projectors connect via an HDMI cable, but many great projectors still use VGA, so it may be a good idea to have both kinds of adaptors so that you can always be sure to connect your laptop.

Know how to calibrate your laptop with a projector

Projectors do not always faithfully display your slides with the same brightness, contrast, hues, and resolution that you see on your screen. In fact, sometimes a projector will not even align graphics on your slides in exactly the same way.

Fortunately, most laptop operating systems contain projector calibration tools that help you match your personal display with what is projected to the audience. You can also use your own calibration slide and observe how it looks just after connecting your computer to a projector. If the slide looks as intended, you can start your presentation. If not, you can use further calibration tools to get your slides looking just right.

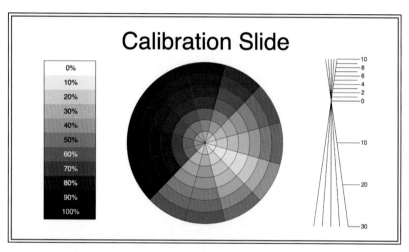

This homemade calibration slide could be inserted into the very beginning of a presentation (before a title slide) to ensure that slides look good before the audience arrives. Surrounding the slide is a red perimeter that ensures that the entire area of the slide is projected onto the screen. At left is a step-wise increase in shades to ensure that whites look white and blacks look black. At center is a color wheel to ensure that all projected colors match their true hues. At right are a series of lines to ensure a good resolution, with numbers representing the number of pixels between the lines. If aspects of this slide do not appear correctly, you can use your laptop's projector calibration settings to fix any problems, or even potentially work with a technical support aide to fix projector settings.

Know how to control your presentation with your keyboard

All slide-making applications feature keyboard commands that let you control your slides during your presentation. Some commands are application specific, but many are common across all platforms. For example, to advance through your presentation, you can hit the space bar, the right or down arrow keys, the return/enter key, or your mouse button. The best choice on a keyboard is often the space bar, as it is the largest key and easy to spot. To go back a slide, hit the left or up arrow keys. To quit your presentation, hit escape.

Two underutilized controls are the B and W keys, which turn the screen black or white, respectively. These keys can be very useful during a pause in the middle of a presentation. For example, if someone asks you a question and you want to draw an answer, press the B key and switch to a blackboard or whiteboard.

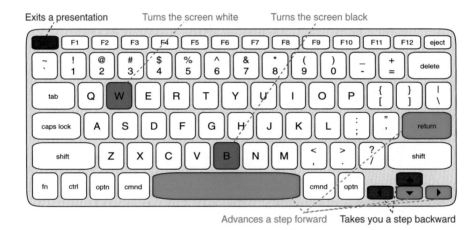

These controls are consistent across all presentation applications. However, there are many more commands you can choose to use. For example, you can use the keyboard to display the cursor on the screen or to control audio and video clips in real time. See the instructions for your presentation application of choice to learn more about the seemingly hidden ways you can control your presentation during a talk.

Use personal display settings to see the next slide

Most slide presentation applications include a special mode that allows you to see something different on your personal display from what is displayed to the audience. This personal display typically includes a preview of the next slide, a clock timing the length of your talk, and presentation notes (if you have any).

While it is usually not a great idea to read presentation notes directly off your computer, a quick, peripheral glance at your screen can provide you with real-time information that will help you improve your transitions between slides and keep track of time. Being able to see the next slide can better help you introduce concepts before you transition to new visual content.

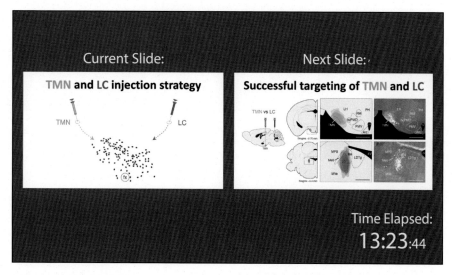

Adjust your display settings so that your laptop screen shows you your next slide and the amount of time that has elapsed.

Learn the light switch before your talk begins

The piece of technology that often causes the most problems during a talk isn't the computer or projector—it is the light switch! Many scientists like to show photographs or videos that look better when the lights are off, but few scientists take the time before their talks begin to learn where the light controls are and how to use them. In larger presentation rooms, light control panels often contain multiple switches and buttons, and it can be confusing to know which ones will dim the room lights in the way you want.

Take the time to learn how to control the room lights before your presentation begins. It is distracting to an audience to watch you play with various light controls that you could have learned beforehand.

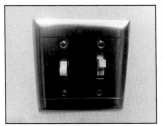 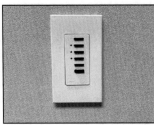 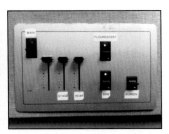

Light switches in presentation rooms can look very different and feature multiple buttons, sliders, and knobs. Take the time to learn how to dim the lights and bring them back up before your presentation begins so you don't have to fiddle around with different settings in the middle of your presentation.

If you can immediately turn the lights off or on without pausing your delivery, your audience probably will not fully realize that you took the time to learn the light switch settings. However, you will seem in command of your presentation and your delivery will be much smoother.

Have a way of keeping track of time

Even if you have rehearsed the length of your presentation, you should have a method for tracking time during your actual delivery. Sometimes the anxiety of talking in front of an audience can make a speaker talk too quickly or too slowly. Depending on the format, audience members may also interrupt your talk with questions, adding time to your presentation. Check out the venue ahead of time to find out if there will be a clock facing you. If one doesn't exist, you can use the timer on your personal display during your talk. You can even bring a small digital timer to face you on a podium that nobody will notice but you.

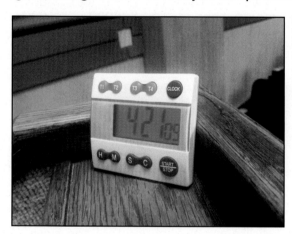

If you don't see an obvious clock in your presentation room, place a lab timer in the corner of the lectern (or another inconspicuous location) so that you can always be aware of how much time has passed during your talk.

Never use your watch to keep track of time. Overtly checking your watch will create the impression that you are bored or counting down the moments until you are done.

It is also a great idea to identify one or two benchmark slides that you should present by a particular time. If you find that you are too far behind or too far ahead, you can subtly speed up or slow down your delivery.

Use a laser pointer to focus the audience's attention

The purpose of a laser pointer is to direct the audience's visual attention to a particular location on a slide. A momentary bright, moving dot is a very salient visual feature that can cause the entire audience to focus on exactly what you want them to see.

Although most institutions will have and provide laser pointers for speakers, consider buying your own (and make sure to bring extra batteries, just in case). Using your own laser pointer will provide familiarity and some degree of comfort during a talk. What color is best to buy? Pointers are typically available in red, green, light purple, and light blue (blue pointers are currently the most expensive—usually $200 or more). In general, green pointers seem to stand out the best against both light and dark backgrounds.

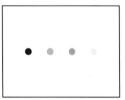 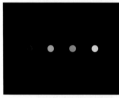

Although red has the highest contrast against a white background and light blue has the highest contrast against a black background, green always has the greatest overall contrast with any background, light or dark.

Some general advice:

- **Use a laser pointer sparingly.** Just like any highlighting tool, the more you use it, the less your highlighted material stands out. Try to use the pointer sparingly so that you only highlight the information you truly want to emphasize.

- **Don't turn the laser on until it is aimed at the screen.** You only want your audience to look at the screen, not a spot on the wall or floor.

- **Don't highlight text.** It is annoying when a presenter reads sentences off a slide while using a laser pointer to highlight each word. If you want to highlight a word, say it.

- **Never aim a laser pointer at the audience.** Even if the pointer isn't on, audiences become nervous at the potential to be blinded at any minute. Consider a laser pointer to be like a loaded gun and only aim it at the screen.

- **Try to leave your pointer on for just a few seconds at most.** Direct your audience's attention toward what you want to highlight, then turn the pointer off. If you leave your pointer on for too long, your audience will stop listening to your narration and will continue to monitor the dot on the screen.

- **If you are nervous, rest the hand holding the laser pointer on your other hand.** This support will prevent your laser dot from nervously shaking around the screen.

Use a remote slide advancer to move more freely

One of the best investments you can make is to purchase a remote slide advancer—a handheld device capable of advancing slides when you are several feet away from your computer. These devices cost anywhere from $20 to $100, and most come with built-in laser pointers (so you don't need to hold two items at once).

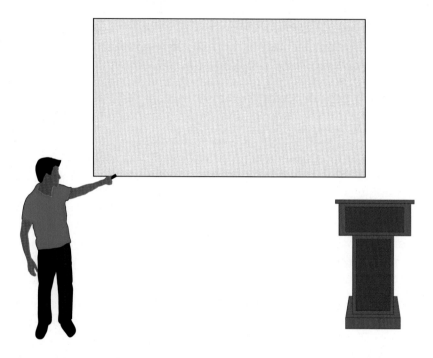

Remote slide advancers liberate you from your computer, allowing you to move freely about the presentation space and better interact with your audience. They also remove the need to constantly look at your computer keyboard each time you want to advance a slide. Instead of making intermittent eye contact with your computer keyboard, remotes allow you to make eye contact with your audience throughout the entire presentation. People who use remotes for the first time often feel like some sort of artificial barrier has been removed between them and the audience, and some even feel that the freedom to walk around the presentation space calms their anxiety.

Considerations for presenting while traveling

Giving a talk while traveling presents you with the extra challenge of adapting to a novel presentation space, often in the few minutes before your presentation begins. In these situations, you should definitely bring your own computer cords, laser pointer, and slide advancer, but you'll have to face the added difficulty of quickly adapting to the new space.

If possible, ask your host about the venue ahead of time. Tell them that you would appreciate arriving in your presentation room 10–15 min before the start of your talk to ensure that you can connect to the projector and calibrate your display settings. If this catches your host off guard, it will only make you look more professional and more motivated to give a great talk. Once you've set up your slide show, find a clock (or set up your own), learn to use the lighting, and settle into your presentation space so that you feel the most comfortable.

Sometimes there are situations in which you will need to present using someone else's computer (such as a conference symposium). In this situation, make sure that you preview every single slide before the actual presentation. If you use any uncommon fonts, they are likely not to show up properly. Also check that all of your media files are present—these files are sometimes not embedded within a presentation itself but linked from a different source on your computer, so they may not show up at all. Finally, be sure to bring a back-up of all of your media files on a memory stick that you can quickly reinsert into your presentation, just in case.

Finally, it is always a good idea to prepare for worst case scenarios. Presenters who are skilled with technology know that technology often fails, sometimes at the worst possible moment. There are various ways to predict and prepare for inevitable moments in which technology fails:

- Bring a back-up of your talk, along with all media files, on a USB memory stick.
- Bring spare batteries for your laser pointer and slide advancer.
- Think of a brief story to share with the audience if you need to stall for time. If you need to restart your computer or a technician needs to fix something, your story will lighten the atmosphere and make you seem like you are in control of a bad situation.

Summary: Design principles for presentation technology

- Learning and mastering presentation technology is the final step in preparing to deliver a slide presentation.

- Make sure to bring your own power cord and any adapters you might need to connect your laptop to a VGA or HDMI projector.

- To ensure that your slides are projected with the optimal brightness, contrast, hue, and resolution, learn how to use the projector calibration tools on your laptop. Reserve a few minutes of time before your presentation begins to calibrate your projection, if necessary.

- Learn the unique controls available to you on your laptop keyboard to control your presentation beyond simply advancing back and forth across slides.

- Use personal display settings on your laptop screen during your talk so that you can keep track of time during a presentation and have a preview of your next slide.

- Learn the location and settings of the light switch in the presentation room so you can immediately dim or turn up the lights when needed.

- Ensure there is a method of keeping track of time during a presentation. If there isn't an obvious clock in the room or if it is hard to see the timer on your laptop display, place a small digital timer on the podium that nobody will see but you.

- Practice using a laser pointer sparingly so that you only highlight the information you truly wish to emphasize. Consider owning your own laser pointer (and bring extra batteries during your talk).

- Consider purchasing a remote slide advancer so that you can move around your presentation space during your talk.

- When traveling, ask your host if you can arrive at your presentation venue 10–15 min prior to your talk so you can ensure that all of the technology around you works properly.

20

Considerations for different categories of slide presentations

Just as different categories of written presentations each have different formats and goals, different categories of slide presentations also have different purposes, inherent structures, target audiences, and optimal methods of delivery. Sometimes the commonly assumed goals of slide presentations are different from what you should actually strive to achieve. Before designing a presentation for any particular category, consider your primary and secondary goals and how you ultimately want to impact your audience.

Designing Science Presentations. https://doi.org/10.1016/B978-0-12-815377-2.00020-2

The research seminar

What it is: An opportunity to share your recent scientific work with colleagues. Research seminars are probably the most formal category of all scientific talks and include invited presentations, keynote lectures, job talks, thesis defenses, etc. The talk typically represents a full scientific story with a clear scientific question, multiple experiments, and a solid conclusion.

Length: 45–60 min (with 5–10 min for questions at the end).

Stated goal: To share your recent work with other scientists and briefly describe work in progress. For a job talk, you will also describe how your previous work leads to future directions in your new lab.

Unstated goal: To establish your reputation as a scientist and make yourself and your work known among the scientific community. Because you can add photographs, videos, stories, and anecdotes to a slide show that you can't add to a formal research article, you can also represent your science in a broader context and amalgamate the results of multiple studies.

Considerations: Because seminars are usually invited by others or required for a job or promotion, they are ultimately the most important category of slide presentation that you can give. If you need to design and build a new presentation from scratch, dedicate many hours/days to ensuring that every aspect of your talk comes across as polished and professional.

When you deliver a seminar presentation, you not only present your science, you also present yourself. Seminars help establish your reputation as a scientist and convey your strategy of approaching scientific problems and finding solutions. If you are a faculty member, your talk may attract future graduate students or post-doctoral fellows to your lab. If you are a graduate student or postdoc, a seminar may earn you a future invitation to apply for a job. No matter what your position, delivering a great research seminar may lead to future speaking invitations, providing more opportunities to meet other scientists and strengthen your reputation.

The panel/symposium talk

What it is: A relatively brief talk grouped with presentations from other scientists about a similar topic. Panels usually occur at scientific meetings and occasionally also among graduate students and postdocs at research institutions (e.g., end-of-quarter rotation talks, senior student symposia). Someone who isn't presenting serves as a moderator of the proceedings and introduces the speakers.

Length: Usually 15–20 min (including 3–5 min for questions).

Stated goal: To share your recent work about a specific topic with colleagues.

Unstated goal: To firmly place yourself and your work within the context of a specific scientific field. A panel presentation is likely to include other scientists within the field and attract an interested audience, and your participation demonstrates that you are a key player within the discipline.

Considerations: Because there are other presentations besides yours, the moderator will strictly enforce time limits. Therefore, you should ensure that your talk is meticulously prepared to fit within the time allotted. You don't have time to figure out how you want to explain your experiments and results on the spot—deliberately plan your explanations ahead of time to ensure that you succinctly describe information in the best way possible. Audience members typically don't ask questions until the end of your talk, so you should be able to develop a talk of a specific length.

Unlike a seminar talk, you might only have time to talk about a single scientific goal or narrow set of experiments. For example, during a seminar presentation you might present three specific aims that all address the same topic; during a symposium, you might only have time to talk about a single aim. It is usually best to talk about a single topic in detail rather than try to cram too many topics into a short talk without adequate time to discuss ideas in detail.

Because panel presentations are usually framed around a specific topic, carefully consider your likely audience and the background material they are already likely to know. If the other presenters and audience members are already familiar with the fundamental concepts and seminal papers in your field, you can omit basic information that the audience already knows and focus your precious delivery time on your own work.

The data blitz

What it is: A special, informal symposium at some scientific meetings and institutional retreats in which each speaker presents a single slide in an extremely short amount of time. Data blitzes usually coincide with poster sessions and allow presenters the opportunity to describe the work contained in their posters in front of all of the meeting attendees.

Length: Usually 60–90 s.

Stated goal: To present your entire research project in 1 min or less.

Unstated goal: To be memorable so that you can have more meaningful interactions with other scientists at a later time. If the data blitz precedes a poster session, another goal is to attract people to your poster.

Considerations: Ignore the stated goal of a data blitz to present all of your work in 1 min. If you do what everyone else does and cram too much information into a single minute, your talk will be forgotten almost immediately.

Instead, simplify your slide and delivery to include only what you want your audience to remember: your name, a one-sentence description of your research, a one-sentence description of why your project is exciting and worth talking about later, and (if applicable) the location of your poster.

Make your single slide stand out in some way. Show a large picture that encapsulates your project or a video that will attract attention. No matter what you do, don't try to cram many figures onto the same slide in an attempt to present your entire project.

Before

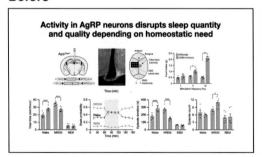

After

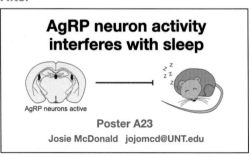

Data blitzes are meant to be fun, but some speakers misinterpret fun as trying to present way too much data at once by talking fast. Instead, try to be memorable so that audience members want to talk with you after the data blitz is over to actually hear more about your experiements.

The lab meeting presentation

What it is:	An opportunity to present work in progress to your labmates
Length:	Varies depending on the culture of your lab: some lab meetings are strictly limited to 1 h, while others can routinely last 2–3 h.
Stated goal:	To share your recent experiments and results with your labmates in a way that solicits advice and feedback.
Unstated goal:	To cement your reputation among your labmates as a careful, detail-oriented scientist who enjoys working as part of a team.
Considerations:	Don't assume that because lab meetings are routine and relatively informal that it is acceptable to deliver a low-quality presentation. Because your labmates give up their time to attend your talk, any lack of effort on your part is disrespectful.

Also don't assume that your labmates are completely familiar with your presentation topic or will automatically remember what you presented during your previous meetings. It is good practice to always start your presentation with a clear description of your scientific hypothesis or goal.

Sometimes people are nervous to present at their lab meetings because they have not experienced good results since their last lab meeting presentation. However, in a good, supportive lab, positive results should never be necessary for a good lab meeting presentation. If you carefully tell everyone the rationale, methods, results, and interpretations of your experiments, they will see that you are a good scientist who might just be experiencing some bad luck. They will also be happy to help suggest ideas for future success. In contrast, lab members don't like it when you avoid talking about your work since the last lab meeting—be forthcoming about how your experiments went and your labmates will be supportive of you.

Lab members like to feel useful. Explain your work in a way that invites feedback and discussion. Try not to act defensively in response to suggestions or criticisms of your work. If you are receptive to the ideas of your colleagues, you will not only improve your own science but you will also communicate to your labmates that you respect their opinions and enjoy being part of a team.

The journal club talk

What it is: An opportunity to present a recent paper (or two or three related papers) to your lab or other colleagues at your institution.

Length: 30–60 min.

Stated goal: To critically examine a recent paper for the purpose of informing others about recent findings or an interesting, novel approach. A related goal is to discuss how the findings or methods used in the paper could directly influence your work or the work of your colleagues.

Unstated goal: To showcase a research topic or method that you are particularly interested in.

Considerations: Don't choose a paper that you aren't enthusiastic about. The best journal club presentations inspire others to do good science and enhance ways of thinking about a scientific problem. It's a much better use of time to inspire an audience with something great as opposed to being a critic of something you don't like.

If the title of your paper contains jargon or esoteric phrases, consider beginning your talk by rewriting the title of the paper in words that your audience can easily understand. For example, in your title slide, write the title of the paper, but then begin your talk by providing a quick translation.

To ensure that your audience understands the context of the paper, it may be a good idea to highlight a few key papers that precede the current study. Although your journal club will be focused on the paper(s) you choose, it is always okay to mention other studies if it helps convey the background and context.

Don't feel that you need to obediently follow the structure of the paper you choose. Although you should highlight the paper's rationale, scientific question, and major results, it is up to *you* to choose what you want to present. Due to time constraints, you may choose only to talk about the most relevant figures. You can also present figures in any order you choose, provided you have good reason.

At the end of the talk, discuss the relative strengths and weaknesses of the paper. Questions you might address include: Do the results of the experiments justify the title? How does this paper contribute to our understanding of a field of science? Are any crucial experiments missing? What are the likely future directions?

The course guest lecture

What it is:	A didactic presentation for an undergraduate or graduate science course.
Length:	Usually 50–75 min.
Stated goal:	To educate students about a topic that is new or unfamiliar to them.
Unstated goal:	To communicate information in a way that students find exciting and memorable.
Considerations:	Many scientists focus scientific lectures exclusively on details and facts that they expect their students to remember for upcoming exams and assignments. However, months and years after the course is over, students will forget almost all of these facts. Therefore, the best lectures also communicate a clear rationale for why the subject matter is exciting and focus on one or two big ideas that students will remember for months or years to come. When you think back to your own college science courses, you probably have forgotten most of the details but remember major concepts, demonstrations, or interesting examples about various topics. Try to deliberately incorporate a "take-home" message into every lecture to highlight one concept for your students to remember after the course is over.

Don't feel like you need to only use slides. Sometimes a slide presentation isn't the best way to convey information, and a whiteboard or demonstration is optimal. Not only is it okay to go back and forth between slides and other teaching strategies, it is also beneficial to student attention. By teaching in different ways, you also reinforce concepts and cater to different learning styles.

Whether fair or not, modern students expect you to post your slides online for future reference. Distributing your slides can pose a problem because, as discussed in previous chapters, you shouldn't necessarily place all of the information you present on your slides. The solution is not to deliberately overwhelm your slides with information just because you want to provide your students with a study tool. Instead, inform your students ahead of time that your slides are not necessarily intended to be study notes. Also consider providing students with a supplementary handout that contains a complete list of the information you expect them to know.

Summary: Design considerations for different categories of slide presentations

- Consider the individual needs of each category of slide presentation. Each type of talk has its own primary and secondary goals for maximal success.

- Research seminars allow you to talk about a major scientific story in a way that you can't achieve in a research article. Because you can add photographs, videos, stories, and anecdotes, you can bring a scientific story to life.

- If you deliver a great talk at a research seminar or panel/symposium, it increases the likelihood that you will receive future invitations to give more talks. Therefore, giving a great talk only increases future speaking engagements and thus more opportunities to meet and network with scientists.

- Make sure that you stick to your designated time limit, especially in panel presentations in which you are one of multiple speakers.

- Use a data blitz as an opportunity to talk with other scientists *after* the data blitz. Don't try to talk too much about your project during the 1-min time limit itself.

- When giving a lab meeting, be very forthcoming with your labmates about successes and failures. Prepare for your talk as seriously as you would for people outside the lab so you don't waste anyone's time.

- Prepare for a journal club presentation talk by choosing an inspiring paper that you are enthusiastic about. The best aspect of the paper you can share with others is why you are enthusiastic and why others should appreciate the science.

- If planning a guest lecture for a course, deliberately think of a specific, take-home message in addition to the facts/details you need to convey. Imagine students remembering your lecture months later and the big picture message you hope they will remember.

Part 5

Designing oral presentations without slides

21

Presenting without slides

As scientists, we are so used to presenting with slides that we don't even notice how protected they can make us feel. When we find ourselves in situations in which we cannot use slides, we can feel naked—as if some safeguard is missing. Indeed, without a screen to look at, the audience will spend most of its time fully engaged in watching you. But this exposure can be an advantage. Although you may feel less secure, presenting without slides increases the direct communication you have with an audience. Therefore, with careful and deliberate preparation, you can use your lack of slides to your advantage to communicate more intimately and effectively.

Designing Science Presentations. https://doi.org/10.1016/B978-0-12-815377-2.00021-4

You never needed slides in the first place

It is easy to forget that scientists have only used slides as visual aids for the previous 30—40 years, and digitally for only the past 20 years. And yet science has, in one form or another, been successfully presented to audiences for thousands of years. Not only did some of history's great scientific presenters (Richard Feynman, Rita Levi-Montalcini, Carl Sagan) not use slides, many exceptional contemporary presenters also use few or no slides (for example, check out online presentations by Jill Bolte Taylor, Richard Dawkins, Malcolm Gladwell, Steven Pinker, and Neil deGrasse Tyson). John F. Kennedy did not use slides to inspire America to go to the moon in the 1960s, and Ronald Reagan did not use slides to convince the nation that human space exploration was still necessary after the *Challenger* disaster in the 1980s.

The key to gaining confidence about presenting without slides is to realize that they aren't necessary or sufficient for a successful science presentation. Successful presentations are more about how you design the structure of a talk, thinking about your audience and conveying the clearest message possible.

Of course, there *is* something missing from a slide-less presentation, and that is a set of figures that communicate the results of experiments. Data are best communicated visually, which is why we prefer to present figures in papers, slides, and posters if we have the opportunity. Without slides, it is more difficult to communicate complex scientific results or compare the quantitative relationships between two or more variables. However, there are tactics to overcome a lack of prepared visual aids. By knowing your data as well as you should, you can develop strategies to communicate results, such as drawing a figure from scratch on a whiteboard or using your hands to draw a virtual graph in space.

The first time you present without slides, you might feel like Dumbo the elephant when he had to fly without his magic feather—yet Dumbo learned that the feather wasn't magic at all and he could fly by himself all along. Likewise, your slides are not magic, and if you feel good about your past presentations, you should realize that your success was due to good organization and structure, independent of your visual aids.

Communicating structure without slides

It is relatively easy for an audience to perceive the structure of a slide presentation: your slides visually communicate the beginning, middle, and end of your story, and if you use a home slide (described in Chapter 14), your audience has a visual roadmap of your entire presentation.

In a presentation without slides, one of the best ways to help your audience is to convey the structure of your presentation using clear, oral statements.

Be very deliberate about communicating the structure of your talk. Also be deliberate about including clear hand gestures that reinforce the structure you convey with your words.

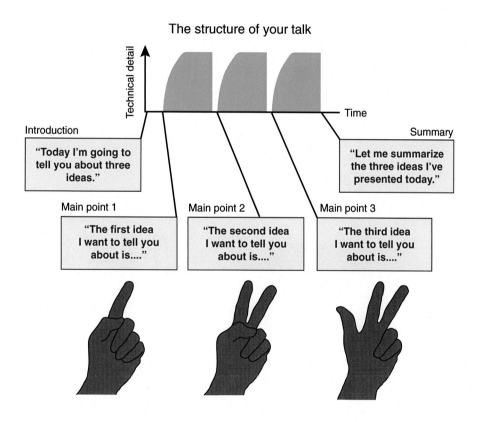

Plan figures ahead of time

For a slide-less presentation in which you can use a chalkboard or whiteboard, just because you don't present a set of prepared visual aids to your audience doesn't mean that you shouldn't design figures ahead of time.

Designing figures for a slide-less oral presentation involves choosing the most important results that you want to communicate, crafting simple figures that are easy to recreate on the spot, and practicing drawing your figures a few times to ensure that you can quickly illustrate them for your audience. Don't forget to practice—you don't want the first time you try drawing a figure to be in front of your audience.

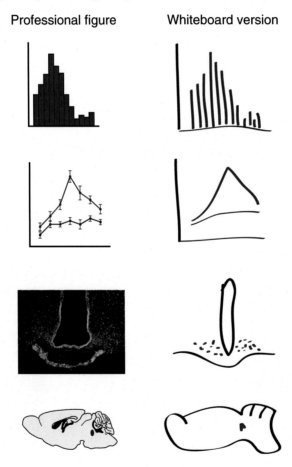

Professional figure   Whiteboard version

Be deliberate about maintaining an audience's attention

Each time you advance to a new slide when giving a slide presentation, your audience members receive a new visual stimulus that can potentially refocus their attention. In a presentation without slides, your audience members only have *you* to look at, and therefore they can become more easily distracted. Although the following strategies for maintaining an audience's attention are useful for any category of live science presentation, they are especially important for a slide-less oral delivery:

- **Maintain eye contact.** If you look your audience in the eyes and keep consistent eye contact throughout the duration of your presentation, your audience will feel more like they are having a direct conversation with you and less like they are passive observers.

- **Smile.** Audiences are more likely to watch friendly, smiling presenters than speakers who seem unhappy to be talking in front of others or who are dispassionate about their topics.

- **Gesticulate.** Instead of keeping your arms at your sides or behind your back, use gestures as much as possible to reinforce what you say verbally and also to be more animated.

- **Ask your audience questions.** If appropriate, deliberately plan two or three moments throughout your talk in which you ask your audience an interesting question: "Does anyone know which planet or moon NASA sent a probe to most recently?" "What are some of the most endangered species on earth?" "What are some of the genes necessary for proper neural development?" Regardless of whether or not you actually decide to solicit answers, asking a question causes your audience members to think about your topic, resulting in a sustained moment of focused attention.

- **Walk around.** Moving objects attract attention more than stationary objects, and in a slide-less presentation the only moving object you can present is *you*. Walking about your presentation space also makes you seem more relaxed and conversational, and provides the impression of an intimate conversation rather than a formal delivery.

Make any presentation notes brief

As for any presentation, you should rehearse an oral talk without slides before your delivery to ensure that you know your material so well that you don't need presentation notes. However, the increased anxiety that might come with an oral presentation can have a powerful effect on your ability to remember all of your main talking points. One of the advantages of using slides in presentations is that if you forget what you planned on talking about next, you can always advance to the next slide to find out. In a presentation without slides you don't have this insurance, and it can be nice to bring notes to help you if you find yourself at a loss for words.

Try to resist the urge to use highly detailed presentation notes during your delivery. The problem with referring to a detailed outline of your talk is that each time you look at your notes, you break eye contact and, potentially, your emotional connection with your audience. Even if you don't plan on consulting your notes and only want to bring them in cause you get stuck, the simple act of bringing them with you might cause you to refer to them more than you planned.

Instead of bringing highly detailed notes, bring a simple outline that is easy to read with a single glance.

Write only a general outline of your talk with two or three main topics and a few "can't forget" talking points for each. Using just a general outline will ensure that you present your most vital information without developing more of a relationship with you notes than you do with your audience.

Before

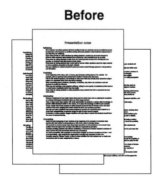

Highly detailed presentation notes are difficult to refer to during a talk without risking breaking eye contact with your audience and interrupting the flow of your talk.

After

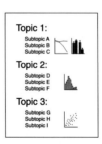

If you decide to bring notes, use a single page with large words in which you can remind yourself of the most important topics with a single glance.

Summary: Design principles for presenting without slides

- Although slides are a great way to visually present information, they are not necessary or sufficient for an excellent science presentation. In situations in when you cannot use slides, it is still possible to deliver a dynamic, clear presentation.

- One of the most helpful ways to design a presentation without slides is to deliberately create a sense of structure for your audience. Use clear, discrete statements and non-verbal gestures to ensure that your audience can clearly grasp the outline of your presentation.

- If you have the opportunity to use a whiteboard or chalkboard, predict the figures you are likely to draw for your audience and practice drawing them ahead of time.

- Because a presentation without slides is not as visually interesting as a presentation with slides, use deliberate strategies to maintain an audience's attention during your talk. Maintain eye contact, smile, gesticulate, ask your audience questions, and walk around the presentation space as much as possible.

- If you bring presentation notes, keep them brief—a single page with large words, so you can access information at a glance.

22

Considerations for different categories of oral presentations without slides

Oral presentations without slides are often less formal than presentations with slides; however, this informality does not imply that slide-less presentations are unimportant or require no forethought. In fact, oral presentations without slides often require more consideration than presentations with slides because you must achieve your goals without visual aids, using oral and nonverbal communication alone. By defining what impact you want to have on your audience and carefully considering the advantages and disadvantages of your specific presentation format, you can design a talk to optimally achieve your goals.

Designing Science Presentations. https://doi.org/10.1016/B978-0-12-815377-2.00022-6

The chalk talk

What it is: A presentation delivered in front of a chalkboard or whiteboard on which you can draw diagrams and charts in real-time in front of your audience, who will ask you questions throughout your talk. The advantage of a chalk talk over a slide presentation is that the audience can help direct the content of the talk in a way that would be impossible with pre-made, ordered slides, and you can adjust your flow as necessary. Chalk talks are often included in job interviews for faculty positions.

Length: 45–60 min.

Stated goal: To present a scientific story or proposal for future experiments while answering a constant stream of questions from your audience.

Unstated goal: To demonstrate that you are exceptionally familiar with your scientific content and that you can think on your feet when questioned by other scientists. If your presentation is part of an interview for a faculty position, you will also be judged on your communication skills and teaching abilities.

Considerations: Although the questions you receive from your audience will require you to be flexible about how you deliver your talk from beginning to end, always thoroughly prepare the structure of a chalk talk as you would for a slide presentation, with a clear beginning, middle, and end. You may have to modify your structure slightly during the actual presentation, but begin your talk with a clear plan in mind so that you deliver a focused and organized story.

Consider writing the major themes of your talk on the board, one at a time, during each segment of your presentation. For example, if you are presenting a proposal for future research and have three specific aims, write each aim on the board as you present it so that your audience will always have a visual reminder of your big picture. Writing these statements is the closest you can come to mimicking slide titles.

Don't face the chalkboard or whiteboard during your talk. When you need to draw something on the board, try to align your body at a 90° angle to both your audience and the board so that you can easily look back and forth between the two while you draw.

The round table presentation

What it is: A format in which a small group of 5–10 people sit around a conference table and each person takes a turn showing the progress and results of their research. This style of oral presentation usually occurs for lab meetings or at annual meetings for awardees of specific grants or fellowships. Sometimes you are asked to bring a brief handout with figures, or you can even bring a laptop or lab notebook with primary results.

Length: 10–15 min per speaker; perhaps 1–2 h for the entire session.

Stated goal: To share, concisely, the results of your most recent research.

Unstated goal: To show that you are making progress on a research project, even if the progress is not in the form of positive results.

Considerations: Although a round table presentation is shorter and more informal than many other categories of talks, make sure that you still prepare and rehearse a presentation with a clear beginning, middle, and end. If you don't have a clear idea of what you are going to say and how you are going to say it, you risk rambling with no coherent message and coming across as not progressing toward a goal.

Just like for any presentation, always state the rationale of individual experiments before you show data. If you bring a handout, wait to pass it out until you clearly explain the purpose and goal of your research. Likewise, don't show data from your laptop or lab notebook until you introduce its meaning and purpose.

Because the energy and attention span of the participants tends to wane over time, usually the people who present first in a round table session speak for longer than those who present at the end. Therefore, if there is no set speaking order, volunteer to present first if you expect to have a lot to say or if you want a lot of attention and feedback from your audience.

The elevator speech

What it is: An impromptu talk in which you give a short synopsis of your research to a scientist or group of scientists whom you have just met, typically in response to the question, "So what do you work on?" The name comes from a hypothetical scenario in which you meet another scientist in an elevator and have only the length of the ride to present a snapshot of your research. This category of talk is quite common at scientific conferences, during which you meet other scientists and only have a brief opportunity to share your work.

Length: 1–2 min.

Stated goal: To effectively and succinctly describe your scientific story and goals to someone unfamiliar with your work.

Unstated goal: To inspire interest and enthusiasm in you and your work and to create a memorable first impression.

Considerations: Just because an elevator speech is spontaneous doesn't mean that it should be unplanned. If you are about to enter a setting in which you will meet other scientists (like a scientific meeting), realize that you will likely be asked to give an elevator speech. Mentally rehearse a short synopsis of your scientific story ahead of time so you are sure to make a great first impression.

A good elevator speech has a similar structure to a good scientific abstract:

- One or two sentences about your overall scientific topic
- One or two sentences about your specific scientific topic
- A single sentence that declares your specific scientific question
- One or two sentences about the methods you use to answer your question
- One or two sentences about what you have achieved so far
- One or two sentences about what you are planning to do in the future

Obviously, you should adjust the content of your research summary depending on the background of the person with whom you are speaking. An expert in the field needs less of an introduction than a scientist from a completely different subfield. In addition to communicating your scientific content, you need to communicate enthusiasm for your work. The more enthusiastic you are, the more memorable you and the content are likely to be.

The speaker introduction

What it is: A short introduction for a speaker before they deliver a longer (usually 30- to 60-min) presentation.

Length: 1–3 min (in general, the more formal the occasion, the longer the introduction).

Stated goal: To provide a brief biography of the speaker for the audience.

Unstated goal: To elevate the speaker's reputation with the audience by highlighting their credibility regarding a presentation topic and establishing why the topic is important and interesting.

Considerations: Most scientists consider a speaker introduction as an afterthought, something that can be hastily put together moments before the start of the talk. This lack of preparedness is disrespectful to the speaker, and often leads to rambling, omission of vital information, and a weak opening to a speaking event. If you are introducing someone who is already well known, you may not feel that the speaker *needs* an introduction; however, he or she certainly *deserves* one.

Establish the speaker's credibility by highlighting key biographical details and achievements such as past research accomplishments, awards, and positions held. Don't mention facts that audiences aren't likely to care about (such as the dates of attendance at universities, or cities where the speaker has lived). In contrast, audiences like to hear specific details about a speaker's accomplishments. For example, you might mention a particularly outstanding research accomplishment and how it led to seminal advances in a field.

Something that most scientists fail to do when introducing a speaker is simultaneously to introduce a speaker's topic. Provide the audience with a strong motivation for listening to the talk and ensure that they understand why the topic is relevant and interesting. The audience will take cues from your introduction, so make sure to convey your own enthusiasm and passion—if you seem disinterested, your audience may become disinterested before the speaker even begins.

Finally, make sure that you get your facts right. Your own credibility and the impact of your introduction are weakened if you mispronounce a key scientific word (especially the speaker's name!) or misunderstand the speaker's research accomplishments.

Summary: Design considerations for oral presentations without slides

- Don't assume that presentations without slides don't require preparation or consideration. Consider the needs of any category of slide-less presentation and deliberately play to the strengths of each format to have a maximal impact on an audience.

- Prepare for a chalk talk by rehearsing how you will convey your main points to your audience. Also rehearse how you will draw figures in real time.

- Prepare for a roundtable presentation by rehearsing how you will explain the rationale, data, and conclusion of each experiment. If you are particularly keen for feedback and advice, volunteer to go first.

- If you are about to attend a scientific conference, prepare for the inevitability that you will have to give an elevator speech. Briefly rehearse a 1–2 min presentation that provides an overview of your research program.

- When introducing a speaker, highlight salient details about the speaker's accomplishments. Also briefly introduce the speaker's topic to prepare the audience for the talk to come.

Part 6

Designing poster presentations

23

The composition of a scientific poster

Poster presentations are the most common way that postdocs, graduate students, and undergraduate students share their unpublished or recently published research. Unlike a scientific talk or written publication, poster presentations allow for personal interactions with other scientists. Because poster presentations are concise summaries of scientific projects, much time and effort is required to explain complicated information as clearly and succinctly as possible.

Designing Science Presentations. https://doi.org/10.1016/B978-0-12-815377-2.00023-8

The purpose of poster presentations

A scientific poster is a large (usually 3 × 4 feet or greater) document that fully presents a scientific story—either a project near completion or a recently published study.

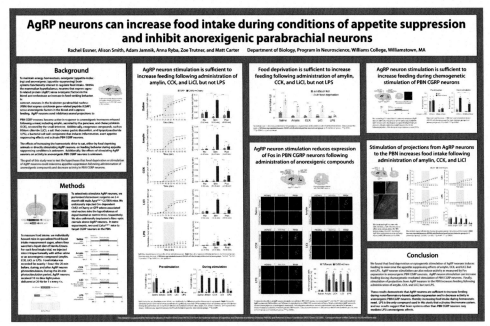

Well-designed posters communicate information visually using minimal text. The more time you spend composing and designing the layout of a poster, the clearer and more impactful your poster will be.

A scientific poster shares attributes of both primary research articles and slide presentations. Like a written paper, a poster contains sufficient text to help a reader understand all aspects of the background, hypothesis/goal, methods, results, conclusions, and other details. Like a slide presentation, a poster allows you to narrate a highly visual presentation with an organized sequence of information. However, a poster has its own major advantage: the ability to interact with your audience through several brief yet meaningful discussions.

The primary purpose of presenting a poster is to meet and interact with other scientists. During a relatively brief 5 min delivery, a scientist can discuss their research, receive feedback, exchange contact information, and then begin a presentation again with a whole new group of visitors.

Posters are presented during poster sessions at scientific meetings or during internal events at research institutions. At large meetings and conferences attended by thousands of people, poster sessions dominate much of the floor space, and many hundreds or thousands of posters are presented at once, usually at the same time as other seminars and talks. At smaller meetings attended by a few hundred people, poster sessions occur separately from talks, and it is theoretically possible for an attendee to observe every poster. At internal retreats, postdocs, graduate students, and/or undergraduates share research with each other at their own institution.

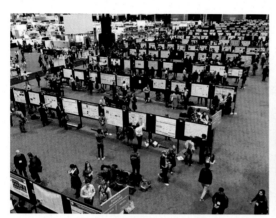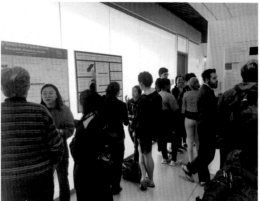

Left, a poster session in a convention center at a conference attended by thousands of scientists. Right, a poster session in a hallway at an institutional research retreat.

Although the ultimate goal of a poster presentation is to interact with other scientists, posters at scientific meetings are often displayed for several hours without the author's presence. For example, a poster session might take place during a dedicated 2-h session, however, the meeting organizers may request that you display your poster for an entire day. Additionally, many authors like to hang their posters outside their lab long after a meeting is over, both to decorate the hallways and also to allow passersby the opportunity to learn more about their work. Therefore, your poster should be able to stand alone so that you don't need to be present for the reader to fully understand your topic.

The best posters are designed both for personal interactions, in which you can refer to the diagrams without reading the text, yet also designed such that a reader can fully understand the poster without your presence.

Because posters are designed to be understood both when you are present and absent, it is important to consider the level of wordiness and detail on your poster. You want your poster to be as detailed and complete as possible so that your audience fully understands your research, yet you also want your poster to be clear, concise, and accessible, without too much intimidating text.

The sections of a scientific poster

The sections of a scientific poster are similar to the main sections of a research article, except that ideally they will only contain a handful of sentences of text. Posters come in all layouts and formats, but they all have a Title, Background/Introduction, several Results sections, a Summary/Conclusion section, and then an area for Acknowledgments and/or References. Sometimes it is optimal to have a Methods section.

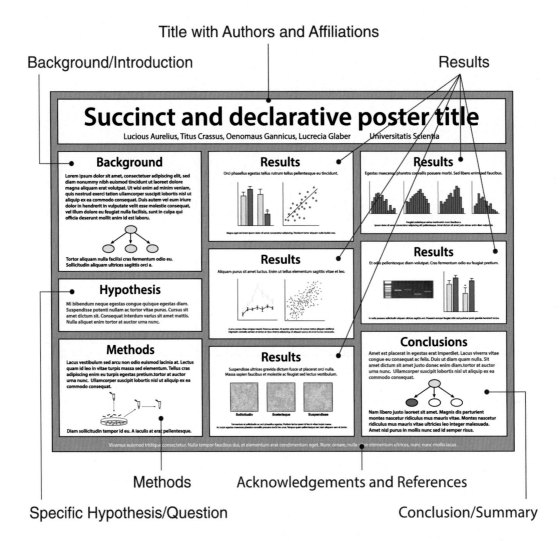

Note that in this example, the text that stands out most is the title, the subheadings, and the red "Hypothesis" and "Conclusions" in red font. By emphasizing this text, a poster reader can immediately distill the key, important details.

The first step: writing an abstract

Usually the first step in presenting a poster is submitting an abstract to a conference organizing committee months before the actual meeting takes place. Once your poster is approved, it is assigned a specific presentation time/date. The meeting organizers will then publish your abstract in an official program so that attendees can find the posters they would like to visit.

Write the abstract for a poster as you would for a research article (see Chapter 10). Most scientific meetings publish an online, searchable program of abstracts. To increase the likelihood that your poster will be discovered by interested attendees, deliberately include keywords in your abstract that someone might enter into a search field. Think of the top 5–10 words that you would want associated with your poster, and make sure that those words appear somewhere in your abstract.

Note that an abstract is not part of the actual poster itself. A poster is essentially already a summary of your research, and if you include an abstract on your poster, you will waste a substantial amount of precious space to summarize a summary.

Never place an abstract on the poster itself. Unlike a research article, your abstract is not part of the actual presentation—it is written for the conference program only.

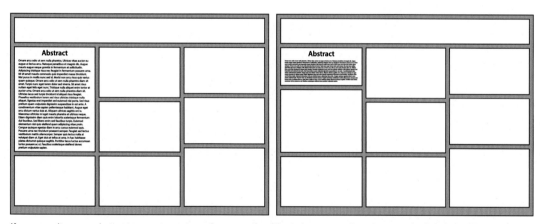

If you rewrite your abstract on your poster using an optimal font size, as on the poster on the left, it could take up a substantial amount of your available space. It is possible to use a smaller font size for your abstract, as on the poster on the right, but nobody will want to read it. And if nobody reads it, why place it on your poster in the first place? Therefore, avoid both of these options and don't place an abstract on a poster.

The best poster titles are conclusions

A poster title is incredibly important because it is the major factor by which a person will decide whether to visit your poster. People searching through abstracts or passing by at a poster session will scan titles to determine which posters to read in further detail. Therefore, compose a title that is easy to read—if your title seems wordy and full of jargon, you will likely turn away potential visitors.

Because poster titles are the one statement that everyone will actually read, they are the ultimate way to communicate your take-home point. Therefore, the best poster titles are clear and specific conclusions.

Before   The effect of stimulating AgRP neurons on appetite following injection of compounds

After   Stimulation of AgRP neurons eliminates the effects of appetite suppressing compounds

Before   Exploring the effects of aromatic ligands on ion emissions in lanthanides

After   Aromatic N-donor ligands serve as chelators and sensitizers of lanthanide ion emission

Before   A survey of factors affecting survival of juvenile pink salmon, *Oncorhynchus gorbuscha*

After   Seasonal food habits are key to survival for juvenile pink salmon, *Oncorhynchus gorbuscha.*

Background/introduction sections should be concise and informative

Your background should provide just enough information for another scientist to be able to understand your poster. In a research article, an introduction might be composed of three to five paragraphs. In a poster, try to limit yourself to four to 10 sentences. Use diagrams instead of words to communicate information and help your reader visualize your topic.

Depending on your content, make it your goal to have at least one visual item in your background section to make this section more visually appealing and to explain information visually.

Highlight your research question/goal/hypothesis

Perhaps the most important part of your poster, other than the title, is a clear statement of your underlying research question, scientific goal, or testable hypothesis. Poster visitors will want to quickly determine the ultimate purpose for why you performed the experiments that follow. Therefore, don't bury or embed this statement in the middle of an introduction section. Either place your research goal in its own section, or call attention to it within the introduction, perhaps using a different font or color.

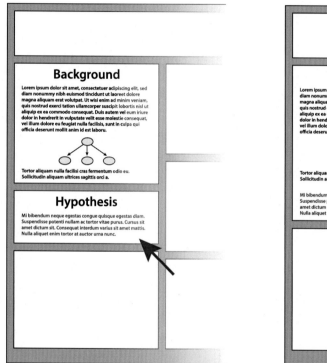 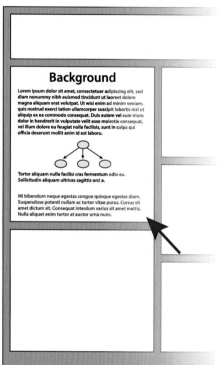

Make sure your hypothesis is brief and stands out in some way. Consider placing it in its own section (left), or highlighting it at the end of your background section (right).

Determine if you need a methods section

A methods section is crucial for a scientific paper, but not necessary for a scientific poster. In a scientific paper, a methods section must have sufficient detail such that a scientist could attempt duplicating your results; in a poster, the main consideration is that your audience understands what you have done. If you used one or two unique methods throughout the entire study, it may be helpful to call attention to them within a single methods section. In this case, consider adding helpful diagrams to visually communicate complex information. However, if you used different methods for each experiment, consider adding a brief statement of methods within each individual results section.

Use results sections to declare major conclusions

Your poster will probably contain four to eight individual results sections, each presenting data that support a conclusion. Don't title these sections "Results"—give each section a specific, declarative title that you will support with your data.

Each results section should be titled with a conclusion, and then the data within that section should provide evidence for that conclusion.

Let your figures do most of the explaining in a results section. To reduce text, write only one or two sentences of explanatory text, and place details about each figure (information about abbreviations, sample sizes, statistical tests, etc.) in a smaller font below the figure.

Before

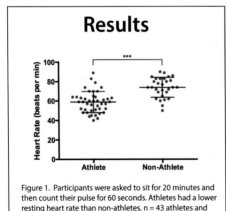

After

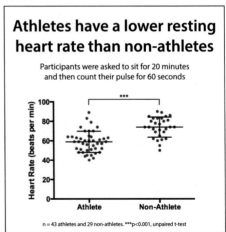

Whenever possible, it is always best to title results sections with the most declarative statement possible based on the data. Add 1-2 sentences about methods or experimental details, if necessary, and then present your data. Beneath your data, in a smaller font, place quantitative/statistical details.

Highlight the major conclusions

A summary or conclusions section is important because it highlights the major points from your study that you want your audience to learn and remember. Just as you highlighted your research question/goal/hypothesis at the beginning of your poster, consider starting a conclusions sections by stating whether your overall research question was answered or whether your hypothesis was supported by your data. Then follow by quickly summarizing the main points.

This section may seem redundant with the rest of your poster, especially if your poster title is already a declarative conclusion about your work and if the titles of your results section are clear about what you discovered. However, readers will appreciate seeing all of your major conclusions summarized together.

At the end of your conclusion, you might end with brief speculation on future directions. Or end broadly by placing your study in a larger context.

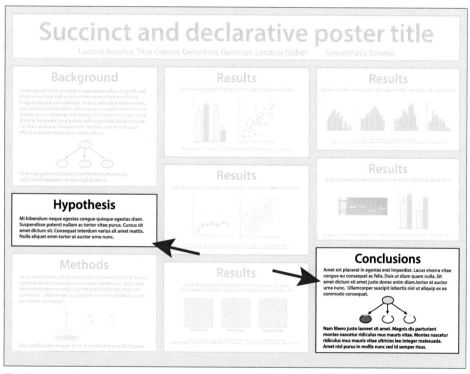

The first part of a conclusions section could state whether the original hypothesis was supported or whether the scientific objective was achieved. To help the reader unite these two sections, write your hypothesis and the first part of your conclusions in the same, distinctive font. Then you can add more supporting statements and diagrams to fully state your conclusions.

De-emphasize acknowledgments and references

Acknowledging your funding sources, as well as the people who shared reagents, equipment, or insightful advice, is important in any science presentation. You may also choose to include citations throughout your poster of key references that are crucial to the background of your study that visitors might like to consult for further information. However, acknowledgments and references can be extremely wordy and distract from the highly visual information on your poster. To de-emphasize the acknowledgments and references on your poster and save room for more interesting items, shrink the font size of these sections compared to the font of the other sections and place them at the very bottom of your poster.

Before   **After**

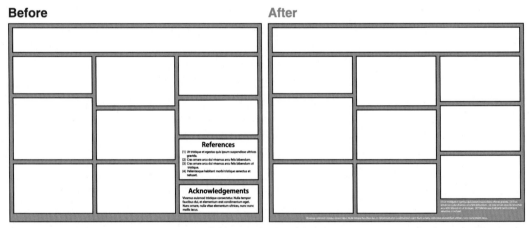

The poster on the left wastes much of the available poster space with acknowledgements and references. The poster on the right includes the same valuable information but minimizes the font size to make room for the much more interesting scientific content.

Reduce the amount of text as much as possible

Although you want your poster to communicate a high volume of information, it is extremely important to compose the various sections of a poster with the least amount of text as possible.

Wordy posters that resemble papers are intimidating to poster session attendees. For example, take a look at the two posters below and ask yourself, as a potential audience member, which poster you would rather read? As an author, which poster would you rather present to a visitor?

Before

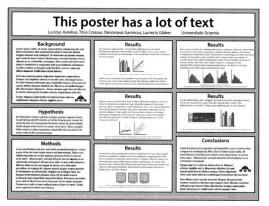

After

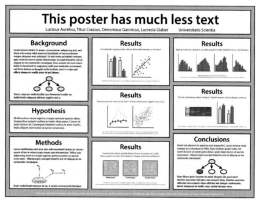

The poster at left is a chore to read and looks like a written document more than a highly visual poster. Potential visitors may be intimidated and walk right by it. In contrast, the poster at right is less intimidating, more pleasurable to read, and easier to present to a passerby. More importantly, the poster is much easier to understand and communicates research much more effectively.

There is an inverse correlation between the amount of text on your poster and the probability that someone will actually read it.

Posters are more like slides than they are like written manuscripts. The goal is to communicate information *visually* with figures and images, not to write a long document that a visitor reads like a paper. The purpose of text is to provide all of the details necessary to understand your figures if you are not present. The total word count for your poster should be no more than 600–800 words. Note that this is 10%–20% of the word count of a typical research paper.

Therefore, as you write the sections of a poster, only include concise information that helps a reader understand your project. Use diagrams whenever possible and minimize the size of text that doesn't convey main points.

Ignore the trend of "Billboard" or "Poster 2.0" posters

In recent years, some scientists have turned toward a trend of designing "Billboard" posters, also referred to as "Posters 2.0." These posters reserve 50%–75% of a poster for a single, declarative conclusion. The rationale is that most posters are poorly designed, and that tired scientists appreciate learning the main, take-home point in a quick, accessible manner. Therefore, these posters attempt to gain the attention of passersby, just as a billboard off the side of the road uses minimal text and pictures to gain the attention of drivers. Instead of displaying results and data, scientists include a QR code with a link to online data.

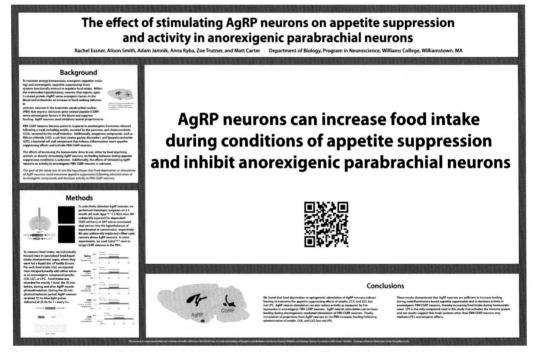

Compare this poster with the poster at the beginning of the chapter. The main feature of this poster, the statement that takes up most of the area, is accomplished in the title of the previous poster. There are no data to provide the basis for interesting discussions with visitors during the poster session. And this poster is uninteresting unless the author is physically present.

These posters are tempting to consider, but they offer severe disadvantages. Losing the ability to share visual data with your audience may prevent meaningful interactions and the ability to receive feedback. Any scientists interested in your data won't want to be referred to a QR code. Keep in mind that the person stopping by your poster may be a future advisor, a future employer, or a future reviewer of your paper or grant. Not showing them your well-organized data is a wasted opportunity. People attending a scientific conference are not like people driving on a highway—they want more than a fast food ad on the side of the road. Furthermore, there is already a place on your poster to display a single, declarative conclusion—the Title!

The best solution to bad poster design is not getting rid of 75% of your poster … the best solution to bad poster design is *good* poster design.

Although the term "Poster 2.0" implies that these poster designs are improvements over traditional scientific posters, they are a trend that will hopefully decline as people realize their limitations.

Advice on composing a poster from scratch

When composing a poster from scratch, it is tempting to immediately focus on the visual design and layout of information. A better way to begin the poster design process is to focus on the structure and composition of your poster, deciding what you want to communicate, what isn't necessary to communicate, and the best order of information. Below is a good, universal set of steps for composing the content of a poster:

1. **Write your specific hypothesis/question first.** Starting with the overall question that drives your research will help you focus on your poster's main message and exclude any content that doesn't matter.

2. **Design your figures.** Spend a good amount of time creating the tables, graphs, photographs, and diagrams that constitute the scientific content of your poster. Your figures are the most important aspects of your poster because they are what you will refer to as visual aids during your delivery, and they are what your audience members rely on to comprehend your work. Designing quality figures is discussed in Chapters 6–9.

3. **Group your data figures into logical categories.** Each of these categories will form the basis of individual "results" sections.

4. **Compose overall conclusions for different categories of results.** These conclusions can then be the titles of the individual results sections.

5. **Arrange your results sections into a logical order.**

6. **Compose a final conclusions section to place at the end of your poster.**

7. **Write your background/introduction section.** By writing the introduction section last, you help ensure that everything you write is relevant to the information you present in your results.

8. **Write a title that offers a succinct conclusion of your scientific project.** If you discover that the title you submitted with your abstract is not the ideal title for your poster, it is usually okay to make slight alterations. As long as your title is similar and you display your poster at the correct time and location, interested visitors will find it.

9. **Design the layout of your poster.** See the next Chapter for advice on the visual layout of a poster. During the layout process, you may need to edit some of your sections slightly so they fit together nicely on the poster. However, writing them before you consider layout issues will greatly help you compose and communicate your scientific story.

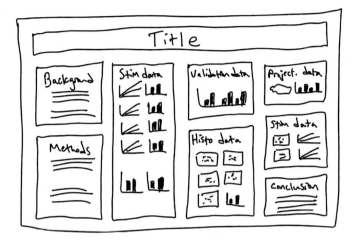

For many people, it is helpful to make sketches of posters before actually creating them. Once you have created your graphs and grouped your data into individual results sections, try drawing them out and determining the most optimal layout before putting your poster together.

Summary: Design principles for poster composition

- Design a poster that communicates information visually to complement your presentation, yet with sufficient text so that the poster can be understood in your absence.

- To attract the largest audience possible and to make your poster more inviting to read, reduce the amount of text as much as possible.

- Submit a poster abstract to a scientific meeting that contains the full story of your project. To help other scientists discover your poster, deliberately include 5–10 keywords that someone might enter into an online search field.

- Ensure that the title of your poster and the title of your results sections are as declarative and conclusive as possible.

- Write a background/introduction section that is both concise and informative, ideally including diagrams instead of words to visualize information and save space.

- To help your reader immediately identify the purpose of your project and how it turned out, highlight your overall research question/goal/hypothesis and also your research conclusions at the beginning and ending of the poster, respectively. Place these items in an individual section, or highlight them using a different font color to make them stand out.

- Only include a methods section if the methods apply to most of the experiments of the poster. Otherwise, include a brief statement on methods within each individual results section to better connect the methods and results.

- Whenever possible, each results section should be titled with a conclusion, along with figures and tables that support that conclusion.

- De-emphasize acknowledgments and references on your poster by writing them in a smaller font size.

24

The visual design and layout of a poster

The quality of a scientific poster is inextricably linked with its visual design and layout. Posters that contain poor font or color choices, meaningless visual distractions, or a haphazard order of information are difficult to read and have less of an impact on audiences. In contrast, posters that present ideas clearly and succinctly in an intuitive, logical way attract more visitors and allow readers to understand information more quickly. Optimizing the visual design of your poster will increase the efficiency with which you communicate information and enhance the impact you have on your target audience.

Designing Science Presentations. https://doi.org/10.1016/B978-0-12-815377-2.00024-X

There are multiple ways to design a scientific poster

One of the most enjoyable aspects of creating a poster presentation is choosing your visual esthetic and layout. What begins as a blank canvas becomes your own unique visual scene.

As you design your poster's visual layout, always remember that your scientific content should be the main attraction. Although you want your poster to be beautiful, your main goal is to clearly and succinctly communicate science. If your poster is well designed, it will be beautiful as a result.

If you want inspiration for the design of your poster, look online. Just type "scientific poster" (or a related term) into a search engine and you'll find thousands of results. Another good place to look for inspiration is the Faculty of 1000 website (http://f1000.com/posters), which publishes scientific posters that were previously presented at conferences. Other sites provide dozens of downloadable templates that you can fill with your own content.

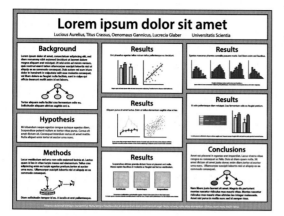
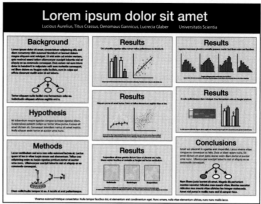
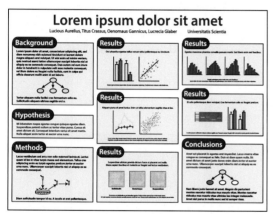
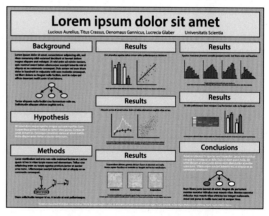
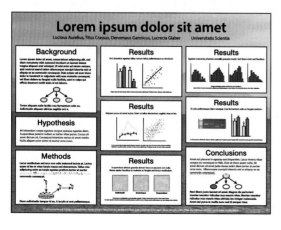
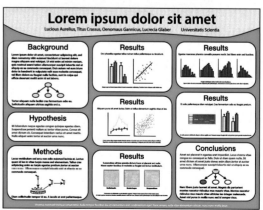

Design an intuitive order of information

Your audience should instantly be able to determine which section of your poster to read first, as well as the correct order of the sections that follow. Unless you have good reason not to do so, it is usually best to arrange the sections of your poster into columns.

Audiences intuitively read the sections of a poster in columns (top to bottom) instead of rows (left to right).

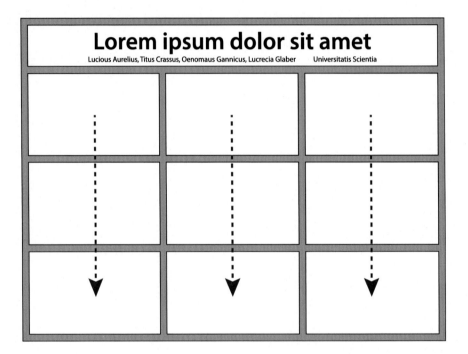

When the natural inclination to read poster sections as columns is disrupted, audiences can become confused about the order of information.

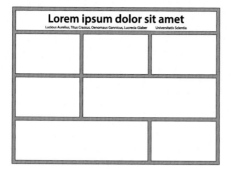 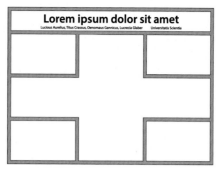

It is possible to inform your audience about the order of sections with numbers or arrows, however, you don't want to make your audience expend mental effort or feel that they have to search for which section comes next. Audiences shouldn't have to do any work to understand your layout.

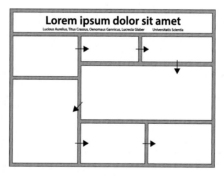

Feel free to play with layout schemes, as long as they follow an intuitive order.

Visually unite the content within each poster section

To help your audience focus on one section at a time, use visual strategies to unite each section within its own border or dedicated space. These visual cues help your readers distinguish between discrete sections and reinforce the divisions between different categories of information.

Creating boxes for each section with different background colors than the overall poster is an easy way to separate the different sections of a poster.

Before

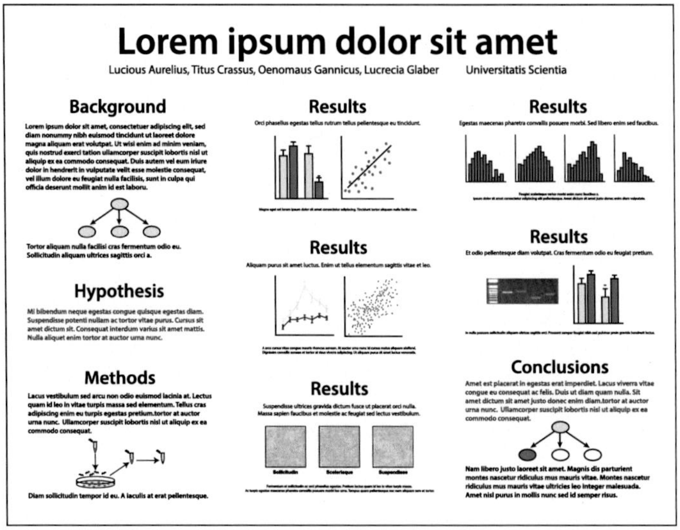

After

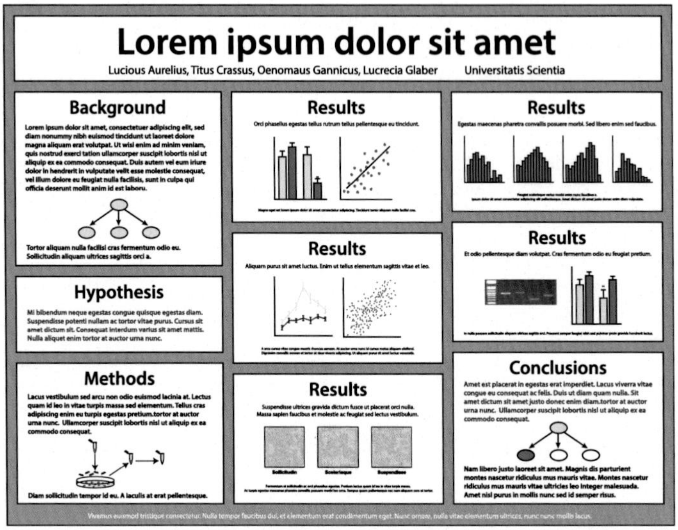

Alternatively, underlining the titles of the various sections (or putting the section titles in boxes) can create the impression of distinct sections.

After

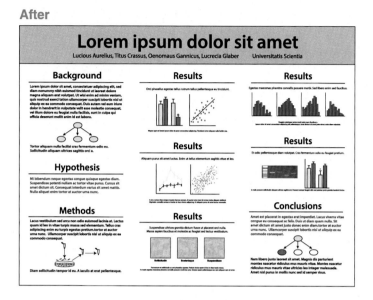

After

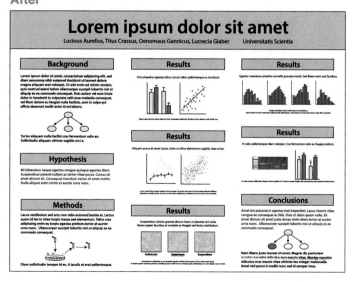

Choose fonts that are easy to read

The principal consideration when choosing a poster font is legibility. Choose fonts that are easy to read and large enough to be seen at a distance.

On posters (as well as other media that are read from a distance, including slides, banners, and billboards), use a sans serif font, such as Helvetica, Arial, Calibri, or Myriad Pro. See Chapter 4 for more about sans serif versus serif fonts.

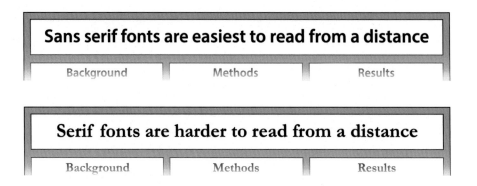

When you decide which font you want to use for your poster, print out a document on $8\frac{1}{2} \times 11$ paper that shows how the font will appear in various sizes. Your poster title should be about 144–256 pts, depending on the font (visible from across a large room). For the main text of your poster, use a font size that is easily visible from 2 to 3 feet away. Smaller font sizes can be used for more specific text that an interested reader will want to examine more closely (such as references, statistical information, etc.), but this text should also be clearly visible from 1 to 2 feet away.

Printing out your own font guides and posting them on a wall will help you visualize how your font sizes will look before the poster is printed. Test out how easy it is to read the various font sizes, both from 1-2 feet away and also from across the room.

If you want to highlight a word or phrase, it is usually easiest to read words in **bold** or *italics* rather than words that are written in ALL UPPERCASE or <u>underlined</u>. The latter options tend to make words more difficult to read and can distract from the rest of the text.

When emphasizing certain words, make sure to **choose a way that is legible**, so that your text is easy to read from a distance.

When emphasizing certain words, make sure to CHOOSE A WAY THAT IS LEGIBLE, so that your text is easy to read from a distance.

When emphasizing certain words, make sure to *choose a way that is legible*, so that your text is easy to read from a distance.

When emphasizing certain words, make sure to <u>choose a way that is legible</u>, so that your text is easy to read from a distance.

Usually it is easier to read the title of a poster in Sentence case (only the first letter of a sentence is capitalized) than Title Case (the first letter of each word is capitalized). And titles written in ALL UPPERCASE are the hardest to read of all.

Titles are easiest to read in sentence case

| Background | Methods | Results |

Titles are a Bit Harder to Read in Title Case

| Background | Methods | Results |

TITLES ARE HARDEST TO READ IN ALL UPPERCASE

| Background | Methods | Results |

Choose backgrounds that aren't distracting

The choices you make about your background colors are important because poor choices can be distracting or even overwhelming. Backgrounds should be just that—backgrounds—that don't overwhelm what is placed in front.

Before

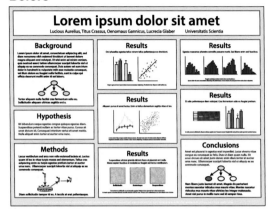 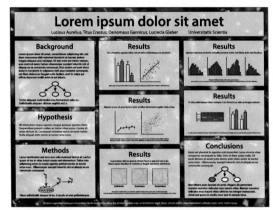

Warm colors aren't good choices for backgrounds because they are bright and can overpower the scientific content in the foreground. Photographs are also poor backgrounds because they are distracting and have uneven light/dark color patterns.

After

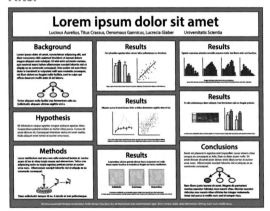 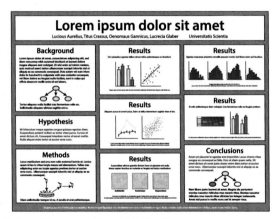

Cool colors naturally fade into the background so that your text and figures are the main attraction.

If you decide to place each section of your poster in its own bounding box, be cognizant about how your text and figures will appear for each background color. If you designed your charts or tables with a white background, it will be easiest to place them on a white surface; otherwise, you may inadvertently create white boxes that can break the unity of the visual scene and introduce an unnecessary visual element. Alternatively, you can remove any white backgrounds from your figures so that they fully blend into the section backgrounds.

Before

After

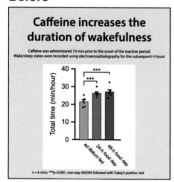 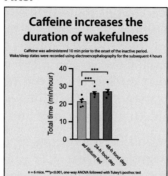 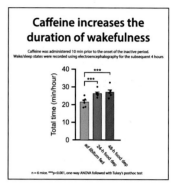

Placing a graph exported from a separate graphing application on a colored background creates the appearance of a white square, an unnecessary visual element. It may be possible to match the green background of the graph to the background of the results section, but it is probably easiest to view the data by removing the green background altogether.

Eliminate extraneous visual elements for clarity

Unnecessary, extraneous visual elements on a poster are not only distracting, they take up precious space that could otherwise be used for your important information and content. Therefore, remove any visual items that don't add meaning:

- **Institutional logos.** Most scientists place these logos on the top of their posters next to their titles, but what purpose do they serve? The authors and affiliations are already located beneath the title. Institutional logos are usually made up of warm colors that can clash with your poster background color and distract from your content. Furthermore, usually scientists feel that if they put a logo on one side of the title, then they need to put something else on the other side of the title for symmetry—so they add another meaningless element, such as the logo of a specific department, a picture of their research subject, etc. It's best to avoid adding logos altogether; doing so will allow you to make your poster title much bigger and potentially attract a larger audience. (By the way, if you ask most scientists why they add logos to their posters, they will tell you that they only think to do it because everyone else does it. That's not a very good reason).

- **Poster numbers.** Once an organizing committee approves your poster, it usually assigns you an official poster number so that your presentation can be indexed in a conference program and cited in future publications. Don't feel that you have to add this number to your actual poster. It does not aid anyone's ability to find your poster, and a number like "Poster AC-0042" doesn't communicate any useful information to your audience.

- **Poster section numbers.** As mentioned previously, readers should be able to intuitively know the order of your individual poster sections without needing a numerical guide.

- **Distracting color choices.** Colors can be used to highlight information, but can be distracting if used in excess. Remember to add design rather than decoration.

Before

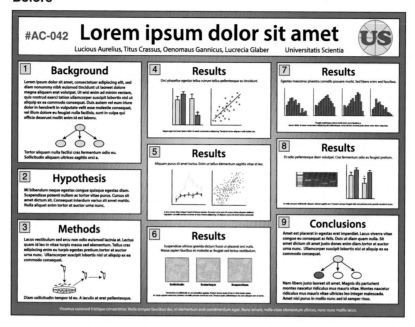

After

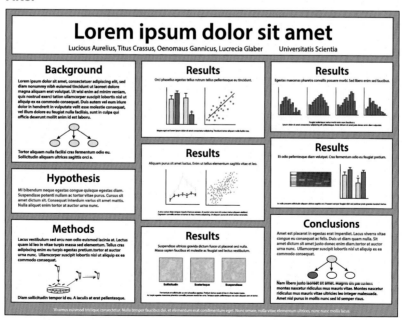

Let your text and figures breathe

Don't be so zealous about increasing your font and figure sizes that you make your poster too crowded. To allow your readers to focus on one element at a time in a way that doesn't feel too busy, surround your text, figures, and even individual poster sections with plenty of white space. In general, the surface area of a poster should be composed of 20%–30% empty space.

Rather than making your poster look desolate, the right amount of spacing between items increases their impact.

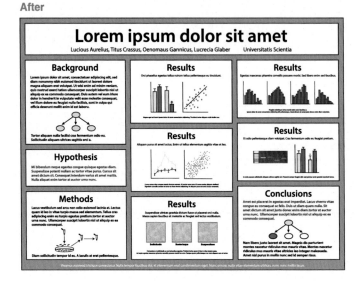

Align visual elements for harmony

The human eye is very good at detecting misalignment and asymmetry, which can create a sense of disharmony and distract from your content. Therefore, be deliberate about aligning the individual sections of your poster.

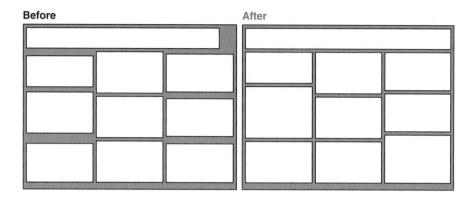

Also be deliberate about how you align text within each box. If you center the title of a section, make sure it is actually in the center. Text within each section that is only one or two lines long usually is easiest to read when center-justified; in contrast, text within each section that runs three or more lines is usually easiest to read when aligned to the left.

Before

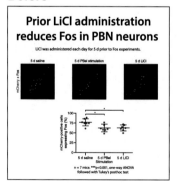

The images seem spaced out a bit too far and the summary graph is not centered beneath.

Before

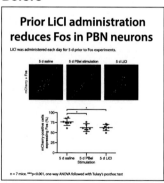

The supporting text above and below the figure is left justified and not centered relative to the data.

After

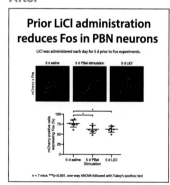

All visual elements are ideally aligned and easy to read.

Choose the right poster printing material

When it is time to print your poster, you will often have a choice between printing on glossy or on matte paper. Most audiences think that glossy posters look more appealing and professional. Glossy paper enhances the color contrast on posters compared to matte paper, resulting in darker blacks, brighter whites, and more brilliant colors. If you have many photographs on your poster (especially fluorescent photographs), glossy paper is always the best choice. The disadvantage to glossy paper is that the gloss can cause glare; however, most poster sessions take place in locations without extremely bright lighting, so glare is often not a problem. Glossy posters are also usually more expensive than matte posters—therefore, if cost is an important factor and you don't have any photographs on your poster, a matte finish may be the best choice.

A third possibility is to print a poster on fabric. Many online companies allow you to upload your poster as an electronic file and they will send you a copy of your poster printed on cloth. The advantages to a cloth poster is that it can easily be folded and transported to a scientific meeting, tucked away with the rest of your clothes! However, there are numerous disadvantages. When displayed on a flat surface, cloth posters tend to hang such that they are stretched and warped in places. When folded in a suitcase, they can accumulate wrinkles that are hard to remove. They also don't provide the same high-quality color contrast as glossy prints or even matte prints. Therefore, it might be best to stick to traditional paper printing, at least for now.

Summary: Design principles for poster layout

- Choose a visual design for a poster that optimizes the scientific content, presenting ideas and data as succinctly and clearly as possible. If your poster is designed to showcase your content, it will be beautiful as a result.

- Design an intuitive visual order of information so that readers know which sections to read in sequence.

- Visually segregate the different sections of a poster in individual boxes or beneath obvious section titles.

- Optimize font choices that are easy to read in terms of font size, color, and casing.

- Optimize the background colors of the poster itself as well as the individual sections to ensure that the scientific content is in the foreground and easy to read.

- To reduce clutter and free up space for more important content, eliminate extraneous visual elements such as institutional logos, poster numbers, and decorative graphics.

- Deliberately add a bit of empty space to your poster to provide your text, figures, and individual poster sections some breathing room.

- Align your text, figures, and individual poster sections for a sense of harmony and balance.

- Choose the poster printing material (glossy vs. matte paper) that is most optimal for your specific needs.

25

Presenting at a poster session

After spending multiple hours composing, designing, printing, and transporting a poster, much of the hard work is already finished. Now it is time to take advantage of all of that hard work and complement your beautifully designed poster with a thoughtful presentation that will allow you to have meaningful conversations with other scientists. Poster sessions are ultimately about interacting with others, and some brief planning and forethought on your part will allow you to optimize the feedback you receive and the relationships you form.

Designing Science Presentations. https://doi.org/10.1016/B978-0-12-815377-2.00025-1

Posters are ideal for interactions with other scientists

Unlike written or slide presentations, poster presentations allow you to meet other scientists, gain insightful feedback about your work, and form meaningful relationships with scientists outside your lab or institution.

Consider that some of the people who visit your poster may be highly influential during the course of your career. Many graduate students meet their future postdoctoral advisors through poster presentations, and many postdocs meet members of faculty search committees. Scientists interested in your work may suggest ideas that lead to meaningful collaborations. Additionally, the scientists who visit your poster may serve as anonymous peer reviewers of your future manuscripts, fellowship proposals, or grants. Therefore, presenting a poster may have profound consequences for your future success, and you should take advantage of the opportunity to meet as many people as possible.

Therefore, maximize the time you spend with your poster audience. If your poster session coincides with a happy hour, skip the food and drinks so that you can concentrate on your visitors. Even if you are only required to stand next to your poster for part of the poster session, try to be present the entire time. If there is another poster you really want to see that is at the same time as yours, try to view it at the very beginning of the poster session. At many poster sessions, most attendees don't start showing up until 10–15 min after the start of the session, so you can use this small window to see some of the other posters.

Anticipate the presentation venue

Poster presentation venues vary in size and atmosphere. Large conferences make use of poster halls the size of airport hangars, where conference attendees navigate through thousands of posters displayed at once. Smaller conferences and institutional retreats may exhibit only 10–20 posters at a time, usually during a happy hour with free food and drinks. Poster sessions also vary by time of day: some start at 8:00 a.m., others start at the end of the evening before social activities.

One of the best ways to prepare for a poster session is to anticipate the likely atmosphere of the venue. Your poster content and design should remain the same from venue to venue, but you may need to adapt your delivery to match the mood of your audience.

Plan to look (and smell) your best

A poster presentation is definitely the most intimate way to present science, as you literally stand just one or two feet away from your audience, likely in a crowded meeting room. Therefore, personal hygiene is key. Bring breath mints, and make sure that your breakfast or lunch isn't stuck in your teeth. Also make sure to wear deodorant but not ostentatious perfume or cologne.

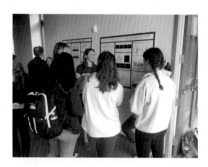

Poster sessions can become very crowded and intimate. Make sure you have impeccable hygiene!

How professionally you should dress depends entirely on the presentation venue. A good rule of thumb is to dress slightly more nicely than your audience. If you are at a professional meeting, business casual is usually best. At an institutional poster session or retreat, you may not need to dress as professionally, but you should dress as you would if you knew your future boss might stop by.

When you stand next to your poster, you immediately become part of your poster's "visual scene." Therefore, wear colors that match or complement your poster's background color, or at least colors that don't clash with your poster's color scheme.

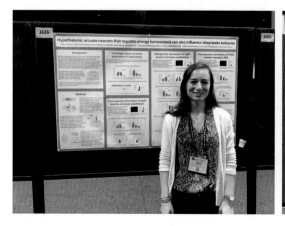

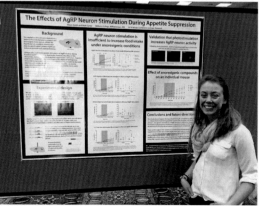

Display your poster professionally

The meeting organizers will provide you with a flat surface and tacks, tape, or a stapler for hanging your poster. Make sure to hang your poster in a way that is aesthetically pleasing and doesn't distract from your content.

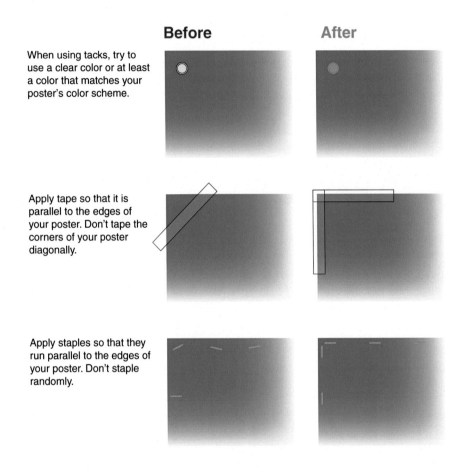

When using tacks, try to use a clear color or at least a color that matches your poster's color scheme.

Apply tape so that it is parallel to the edges of your poster. Don't tape the corners of your poster diagonally.

Apply staples so that they run parallel to the edges of your poster. Don't staple randomly.

At larger meetings, your poster will almost certainly be assigned a specific location (so it is easy for interested visitors to find). At smaller meetings, posters may be displayed on a "first come, first served" basis, with presenters hanging their posters wherever they find space. If this is the case, try to display your poster near an area of higher traffic—such as an entrance/exit, a drinking fountain, etc. Try to avoid areas of low traffic and where the environment may repel visitors, such as near a noisy air vent.

Prepare for potential problems with a poster repair kit

Although you proofread the final version of your poster multiple times before printing, there is nothing like displaying your full-size poster at the actual venue to make you realize an embarrassing error. For this reason, it is great to bring a small kit to quickly fix your mistake and any other rips or tears that may occur during transport. Items to bring include pens with the same color as the fonts you used, a small bottle of correction fluid or "white tape," a small cloth to wipe away fingerprints (especially for glossy prints), and clear tape to fix any rips or tears. If you have to use tape, be sure to tape the *reverse* side of the poster and not the side your audience will see.

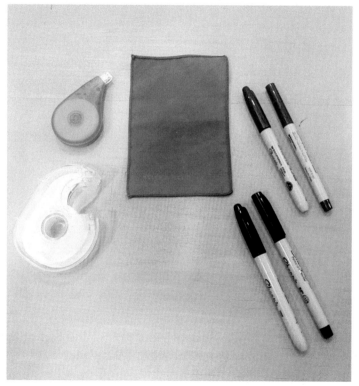

The contents of a modest poster repair kit.

Be deliberate about being friendly and approachable

Although communicating enthusiasm to your audience may seem obvious, even the perkiest of personalities can become tired after a multi-hour poster session, or especially during periods in which few or no visitors stop by your poster (which is inevitable, and happens to everyone at some point!). If nobody stops by your poster, resist the temptation to walk away or check your email. Showing disinterest in your own poster or future visitors will only cause you fewer visitors in the future. As hard as it may be, try to remain by your poster looking outward, friendly, and happy to talk with anyone passing by.

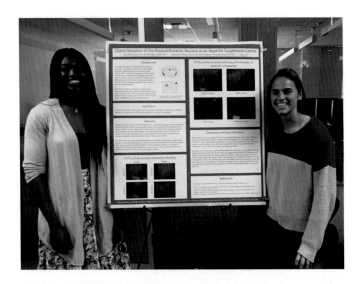

You will attract many more visitors if you make eye contact, smile, and appear happy to talk about your poster.

Speak to your audience as you walk through your poster instead of looking at notes, poster text, or your watch. Keep your hands out of your pockets, as this conveys a lack of enthusiasm. **Never look at your phone**.

Finally, at a scientific meeting, wear a visible nametag with your first and last name. Approaching visitors want to know who is talking, especially if you are one of the authors listed on the poster. Visitors may also recognize your name if you recently published a paper of interest.

Present your poster by giving a brief "walkthrough"

A walkthough is a brief guided tour of your poster for interested visitors. It is essential that you keep your walkthrough as brief as possible.

Keep your walkthrough to 5 min or less. If individual visitors want more explanation, they will let you know by asking follow up questions. If you go on too long, they will be polite, but silently wish they were somewhere else.

To ensure a short delivery, you should plan what you are going to say in advance and mentally rehearse before visitors arrive. The following is a good, generic walkthrough for most posters:

- Introduce yourself and your research interest: "My name is Matt and I'm interested in ..."

- Provide a brief introduction (two or three sentences): "The physiological basis of xxx is unknown. Previous studies have demonstrated A, B, and C, but D is unknown. The goal of my research is to study D."

- If relevant, provide a brief explanation of the methods you used.

- Describe each result as its own mini-study, with a rationale, statement on methods, statement on results, and conclusion. "We first decided to examine ... To investigate, we ... We found that ... This result means that ..."

- Summarize the two to four main conclusions of your study.

- Provide a brief statement about future directions.

- ***Thank your visitors*** for stopping by your poster. And be genuine—your visitors could have spent their 5 min doing something else.

If additional visitors arrive halfway into your walkthrough, make sure to finish your presentation for your current audience first before starting from the beginning.

During your walkthrough, point to the various figures on your poster to show your data, but don't point to text. The information on your poster should be the same as the information that you say out loud.

Also, let your narration lead you through your figures rather than letting your figures lead your narration. Discuss your concepts and point to figures for support, rather than pointing to figures and then explaining the concepts behind them.

Know where you stand

Try not to block your poster by standing in front of it—a common beginner's mistake. When greeting new visitors, stand to the left of the poster. At some point, as you describe the various sections to your visitors, completely cross to the other side and remain there until you thank your visitors for stopping by. Finally, walk back to the left side of your poster again to start over with a new group of visitors.

Always start a walkthrough by standing just to the left of your poster.

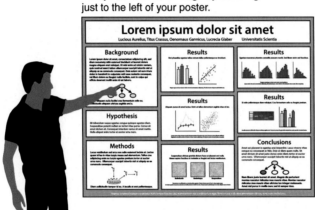

When you are about halfway through, completely cross to the other side.

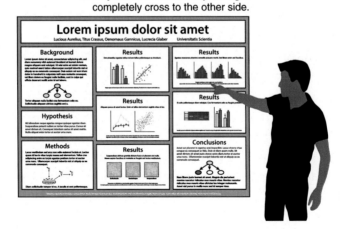

Providing supplementary information

Consider bringing miniature versions of your poster that visitors can take as handouts. If you have prior publications that are relevant to your poster, you can also bring along reprints for anyone interested. Keep in mind that poster session attendees generally don't like being given items to carry around with them, so only offer handouts if someone seems genuinely interested.

Just as research papers can include supplementary movies and figures, you can also provide supplementary materials for your poster. For example, if a short video will easily convey information to your visitors, bring a tablet computer or mobile phone to show your video to anyone who is interested.

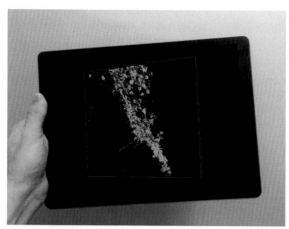

A tablet or smartphone is a great way to show additional movies, animations, or 3D models to poster visitors.

If relevant, embrace the senses and think of ways to share sounds, smells, textures, or even tastes with visitors. For example, if you study bird song, offer to play a 5–10 s clip of song recordings to your visitors. If you study how mice respond to odors, bring examples of the odorants in small vials or bags. Audiences appreciate these kinds of "show and tell" moments, and you might attract a bigger crowd.

Summary: Design principles for presenting a poster

- After spending many hours composing and designing a poster, complement your hard work by also being thoughtful about the poster presentation itself.

- To prepare for the intimate atmosphere of the poster presentation session, dress professionally in a way that complements your poster design, and look and smell your best.

- Display your poster as professionally as possible and prepare for potential mistakes, rips, or tears with a homemade poster repair kit.

- Attract visitors to your poster by presenting yourself as friendly and approachable as possible. In between visitors, smile at passersby and never look at your smartphone.

- Plan a succinct walkthrough of your poster that lasts no longer than 5 min. If individuals want more explanation, they will ask follow-up questions.

- Never stand in front of your poster—always stand just to the left or righthand sides.

- Be creative about providing relevant supplementary materials—handouts (if requested), reprints of papers, movies on mobile phones or tablet computers, sensory handouts, etc.

Appendix 1

Recommendations for further reading

Quite a few books have inspired me in my own presentation design. The following seven books continue to have a profound influence on the way I design science presentations and I recommend all of them very highly.

Books about universal design principles

Universal Principles of Design: 125 Ways to Enhance Usability, Influence Perception, Increase Appeal, Make Better Design Decisions, and Teach through Design by William Lidwell, Kritina Holden, and Jill Butler.

Concise, well-written, and completely accessible, this book is a design course for people who have never taken a design course. These 125 principles not only inform the creation and delivery of visual information, they also teach problem solving, innovation, and creativity. I honestly think I learned something from every single page.

100 Things Every Designer Needs to Know About People by Susan M. Weinschenk.

A highly visual and accessible book focused on design thinking for human nature. As mentioned throughout this book, one of the most important design goals is to know your audience and to make decisions with them in mind. This book has greatly helped me think about audiences and to deliver information that is most likely to resonate.

Books about science/data presentations

The Craft of Scientific Presentations: Critical Steps to Succeed and Critical Errors to Avoid by Michael Alley.

The most appropriate word in the title might be "craft," because this book is truly about developing a set of skills necessary to design and deliver exceptional science presentations. Alley reflects on contemporary and historical science presentations, translating other scientists' successes and failures into practical and useful advice.

The Visual Display of Quantitative Information by Edward R. Tufte.

A modern classic on the design of data graphics. Tufte examines the creation of charts, tables, and diagrams from the point of view of a designer, describing how to discard nonessential "chartjunk" and only include what is necessary to convey meaning.

Better Presentations: A Guide for Scholars, Researchers, and Wonks by Jonathan Schwabish.

One of the few books on scientific presentation design written directly for researchers and academics instead of for people in business and marketing. A very visual guide that is especially good at describing presentations involving data.

Books about slide presentation design

Presentation Zen: Simple Ideas on Presentation Design and Delivery by Garr Reynolds.

This book provides a very beneficial and unique perspective on making slide presentations, combining principles of design with the tenets of Zen simplicity. It doesn't merely describe how to create and deliver good presentations, it re-imagines the way you should think about presentation design: as a journey of simplicity, wisdom, and truth. Every time I pick up this book, I wish I was at the beach… with my laptop!

Slide:ology: The Art and Science of Creating Great Presentations by Nancy Duarte.

Slide:ology is a highly visual textbook about story development, inspirational design, and creating exceptional, dynamic slides. Throughout the book, Duarte includes many examples of slide and presentation design from the world's best speakers and leading brands. I continually flip through this book for inspiration.

Appendix 2

Using illustration and presentation software

Throughout this book, I recommend guidelines for creating figures and presentations while deliberately avoiding any description about using modern illustration and presentation software. If this book were to provide step-by-step advice about how to use computer applications, it would be about five times as long. However, I am often asked which applications I use and how I learned to use them.

Personally, I only use five applications to create all of my science presentations:

- Word (Microsoft)
- Keynote (Apple)
- Photoshop (Adobe)
- Illustrator (Adobe)
- Prism (GraphPad)

These are not necessarily recommendations, although I do enjoy using these programs. Actually, I will go ahead and highly recommend Prism as a statistics and graphing program. The user interface is very intuitive, and the default graphs are terrific. Furthermore, it is easy to change elements in each graph to a style of your liking and even export the graphs to Illustrator for further figure creation.

For slide presentations, I used to believe that Keynote was far superior to PowerPoint for making presentations, however, I think PowerPoint has matured and they both seem great. I have equal numbers of colleagues who choose to use Keynote or PowerPoint, and I've seen equally great presentations from both. Many of my students are now using Google Slides, and they also deliver great talks. I'm not a fan of Prezi... if ever there was an application that violates the rule of "let the content be the star," it is Prezi, which deliberately distracts audiences with flashy slide transitions and unnecessary backgrounds.

Although I don't have any formal training in graphic design or visual arts, I feel confident in my ability to create any figure or presentation that I want. I learned how to use Photoshop and Illustrator in graduate school, partially on my own, partially by skimming some guidebooks, and partially by looking for answers to my questions on the internet. Additionally, throughout my career, the academic institutions I've worked at all offered short workshops and courses on how to use these applications. There were many opportunities to learn, and I just had to be proactive about taking them. If I need to make a diagram to realistically depict a real object (e.g., a piece of equipment, an animal, a research specimen, etc.), I scour the internet for good photos to use as source material. Then I create a "cartoon" version using Illustrator.

If you feel deficient in using the applications mentioned above (or other applications of your choice), realize that these are tools you can learn on your own in a short amount of time. There are many wonderful step-by-step guidebooks that describe how to use all of these programs. Many of these books are written in a "lesson in a day" format so that you can teach yourself a useful function in just 30–60 min each day. I taught myself how to use all of the programs above in just a few weeks (usually while waiting for gels to run or DNA to fully flow through purification columns). Also, the mighty internet has never failed to answer any of my specific questions when typed into a Google search field (e.g., "How do I create an opacity gradient in Illustrator?").

In short, don't be intimidated by presentation technology. The software engineers really have done a remarkable job making these applications fun and simple to use. Some minimal effort, complemented with a good guidebook or workshop, is really all that you need.

Appendix 3

Thoughts on how to design
a presentation from scratch

Many people find that the hardest part of designing a science presentation is starting. True, when you begin working on a written, slide, or poster presentation, there isn't anything quite as intimidating as a blank screen. For many years, I forced myself to stare at these blank screens until I was finally able to type something, but this was a miserable process, and not only did I not have fun, I wasted a lot of time. Only recently have I figured out a more efficient process that makes the design and creation process more fun and efficient. While these methods might work better for some than others, I offer four pieces of advice for designing presentations from scratch:

1. **Start by keeping your computer closed.** Adding information to a page or slide before determining what you want to say is like getting into a car before you know where you want to drive. I don't open my computer until I have a pretty good idea of what I am about to do. If I find myself stuck, I close my computer again and don't come back until I have a new plan. If you feel yourself staring at a blank screen for several minutes, walk away. Your computer will be waiting for you when you come back with a new idea.

2. **Create an outline before you start working.** It is always best to have a roadmap for your presentations before you begin. If you are writing a paper, you should initially determine the theme and order of your figures and the title of your figure legends. If you are creating a slide presentation, you should outline the beginning, middle, and end of your talk. If you are composing a poster, you should determine what each section will be about. Because it is difficult to keep track of all of this information in your head, you might consider a method of visually recording your ideas. I like to sketch my ideas on scratch paper or a whiteboard. Other people like to use sticky notes or index cards. It doesn't matter what you use as long as you can see all of your ideas in front of you. After writing everything out, I start to group similar content together and eliminate the information that doesn't seem to relate to anything else.

3. **Take brainstorming breaks while moving around.** Go for a walk. Go for a hike. Take a shower. Everyone has their own personal space for coming up with good ideas. For whatever reason, most people think better when they are standing or walking than when they are sitting. I don't know a good reason why this should be true, but for me, it is a fact of life. My best ideas, scientific and otherwise, come to me while standing in line for coffee, walking to work, or mowing the lawn. For many years now I've applied this self-realization to designing science presentations. When I need to come up with a new section of a paper, slide show, or poster, I always go for a quick walk. Sometimes I bring a clipboard with me so that I can write down good ideas along the way. (Here's a little secret I'll share with you at the end of this book: most of the first draft of this book was written while walking.) Only after I brainstorm ideas and go for a quick walk do I return to my desk and turn on my computer. The screen may be blank, but I fill it with content within minutes.

4. **Deliberately write each section one piece at a time.** It is so intimidating to open your computer with the thought "I need to write a paper," or "I need to design a new talk." Those intentions can make designing science presentations seem insurmountable. Instead, deliberately plan to compose a presentation one piece at a time. Go to a coffee shop and tell yourself your entire goal will be to write a first draft of a methods section. First thing in the morning after you get to work, write one more paragraph of your introduction or compose a few new slides of your upcoming talk. Writing one piece at a time not only makes designing a presentation less stressful, it makes designing more fun because you can spend longer brainstorming individual chunks. And accomplishing more goals makes you feel like you are being more productive.

Whenever I give talks about science presentation design, I always end with the same final piece of advice: Have fun! Designing a presentation from scratch is hard work, and it is much more enjoyable the more fun you are having. Give yourself license to try new ideas, make mistakes, and to continually improve. As mentioned in the first chapter, declaring a science presentation finished is not the same thing as declaring a science presentation perfect. Try your best, and have fun doing it!

Index

Index

Index

Index